ACUPOINT TAPPING

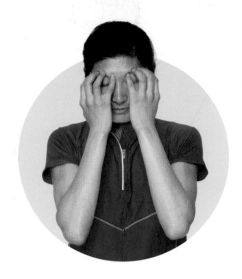

Copyright © 2014 Shanghai Press and Publishing Development Company
Chinese edition © 2012 Chemical Industry Press

This book is edited and designed by the Editorial Committee of *Cultural China* series

Text by Huang Guangmin
Exercise Demonstration by Xing Huina
Translation by Cao Jianxin
Cover Design by Wang Wei
Interior Design by Yuan Yinchang, Li Jing, Hu Bin (Yuan Yinchang Design Studio)

Assistant Editor: Hou Weiting
Copy Editor: Kirstin Mattson
Editors: Yang Xiaohe, Wu Yuezhou
Editorial Director: Zhang Yicong

Senior Consultants: Sun Yong, Wu Ying, Yang Xinci
Managing Director and Publisher: Wang Youbu

ISBN: 978-1-60220-016-6

Address any comments about *Acupoint Tapping: A Natural Way for Prevention and Treatment through Traditional Chinese Medicine* to:

Better Link Press
99 Park Ave
New York, NY 10016
USA

or

Shanghai Press and Publishing Development Company
F 7 Donghu Road, Shanghai, China (200031)
Email: comments_betterlinkpress@hotmail.com

Printed in China by Shenzhen Donnelley Printing Co., Ltd.

1 3 5 7 9 10 8 6 4 2

ACUPOINT TAPPING

A Natural Way for Prevention and Treatment
through **Traditional Chinese Medicine**

Huang Guangmin

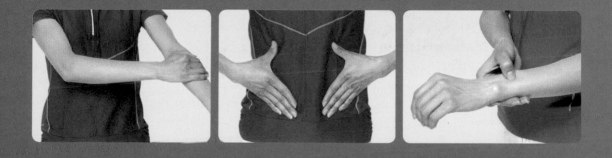

Better Link Press

Contents

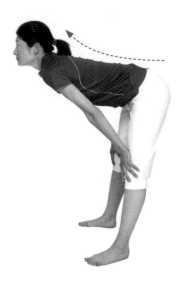

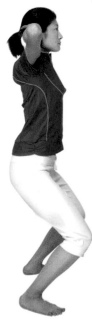

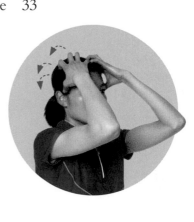

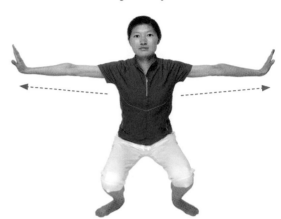
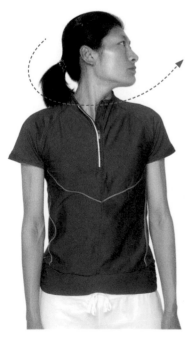

FOREWORD

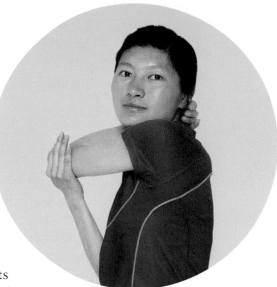

Stretching your arm around your neck and grasping your ears can prevent periarthritis of the shoulders and cervical degeneration.

I experienced benefits from these special exercises of tapping meridians and collaterals the very first time I practiced them, during one of our institute's activities.

Following the oral instruction of Mr. Huang Guangmin of the Institute of Sports Medicine at China's General Administration of Sport, a group of us practiced these exercises, and felt much more comfortable from head to toe afterward. In my professional opinion based on ten years of experience in the public health field, this set of exercises is simple, convenient and practical. It is not only suitable for middle-aged and elderly people but also busy office workers.

Mr. Huang looks like a middle-aged gentleman. While listening to him introducing his own experience, I found that the years he mentioned disagreed with the age he appeared to be. Therefore I boldly asked him how old he was. His answer amazed me considerably. He turned out to be more than 60 years old. I could not help wondering, "How has he managed to appear so young, hale and hearty?"

This mystery was not uncovered until I accompanied him to Qingdao for another activity. While waiting for a train, other people might try to find a seat in the waiting room. Instead Mr. Huang put his luggage on the ground and walked around it, patting his arms in turn. After walking around the luggage more than ten times, he stood in front of it and began to practice acupoint tapping up and down his body, as calmly as if there was no one else present.

After sitting down in the train, I asked him curiously, "Your physical condition and spiritual state are quite inconsistent with your actual age. Can it be attributed to this set of tapping exercises?" He answered, "Yes. However the most important thing of all is not the exercises themselves, but how to consciously use your spare time to exercise your body and keep fit at any time and any place."

These methods provide a clear way toward better health, but only sticking to them can produce a desirable effect.

Chen Dongniu
Director of Beijing Sunshine Public Health Research Institute

PREFACE

This book explores ways in which you can use simple methods to tap, or manipulate, certain key points on your body to improve and maintain your health. These methods are based on traditional Chinese medicine's system of meridians and collaterals, which are special channels that together form a network for the circulation of blood and qi. Using this approach can empower you to control your own health.

Tapping can clear the meridians and collaterals of the whole body, strengthen the body's resistance, and coordinate functions of various internal organs. These methods are suitable for a diverse group of people, from patients with chronic diseases and those in a sub-optimal state of health, to healthy people who need to maintain and reinforce their health and prevent diseases. You can choose an individualized program of treatment according to the state of your health.

Chapter One of this book will introduce methods of tapping meridians and collaterals. These methods require only the use of your hands or simple instruments. The whole body is patted, following a specific sequence and route, although you can benefit without memorizing acupuncture points. For easy mastery, I will introduce these methods in order from the easiest to the most difficult: tapping parts of the body; tapping specific meridians and collaterals; and tapping meridians and collaterals of the whole body.

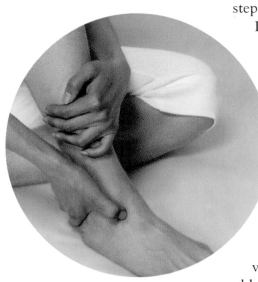

Pinching and rubbing the Qiuxu point can treat insomnia.

Chapter Two will introduce a sequence of sixteen steps, or exercises, of the meridians and collaterals. In practicing the exercises, channels or acupoints are stimulated through such techniques as pinching, rubbing, dredging, scraping and patting, thus clearing all of the body's meridians and collaterals.

These exercises regulate some of the basic forces in traditional Chinese medicine (TCM). First, they regulate the balance between yin and yang. According to TCM, yin and yang are the two fundamental principles in nature, which are present in everything in the natural world. They also regulate the flow of qi (the vital energy, or life force, of the human body) and blood, invigorating the body and strengthening its resistance to pathogenic factors. In terms of Western medicine, the exercises can improve cardiovascular function, adjust blood pressure and increase heat energy consumption by regulating the functions of internal organs.

Meridian and collateral exercises are flexible, and can be practiced anywhere from just a few minutes to an extended period of time. However when time allows, it is best to practice the whole set of exercises to achieve the most complete effect. The exercises can be done at different times of day: in the early morning, during work breaks, in the afternoon, in the evening or at night. Keep in mind that you should wait thirty minutes after meals, to eliminate any harm to the spleen and stomach.

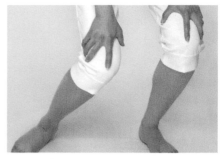
Knee and ankle rotation helps to enhance flexibility of the joints.

Chapter Three, Chapter Four and Chapter Five of this book offer a complete set of solutions for a range of health conditions, with some for the healthy group, others for the ten types of sub-healthy people, and for those suffering from nineteen chronic diseases. These prescriptions include:

1. Recommended exercises: Based on one's physique and symptoms, the most relevant methods can be chosen from among the sixteen set of exercises introduced in Chapter Two.

2. Self-massaging suggestions: To complement the exercises, massaging of different acupoint combinations is prescribed according to specific physical states.

3. Other tips: Certain sports and modifications to daily behaviors are recommended based on health state.

In additional to requiring no expensive equipment, the methods introduced in this book are simple and easy to learn, and suitable for people of different sexes and ages. Everyone will be able to feel the positive effect of practicing these methods, and in growing to trust and appreciate them, each individual will gradually develop his or her own habit of using these methods. This will allow you to become a qualified protector of your own health, and improve your quality of life.

By practicing these exercises, healthy people can become healthier, and sub-healthy people can gradually say goodbye to illness. For those suffering from diseases, practicing these exercises in combination with medical care can help patients meet their urgent needs, relieve symptoms, aid their therapy and recuperate their health.

It is a great honor for me that Xing Huina, gold medalist in the 10,000 m race at the 2004 Athens Olympic Games, has posed for more than 100 action photos for this book. I would like to express the most sincere gratitude to Xing Huina, and invite you to follow us to better health!

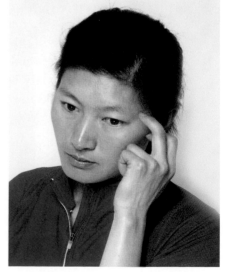
Massaging your Taiyang point is good for your eyes.

INTRODUCTION

I n traditional Chinese medicine, healthcare focuses on protecting health with a particular emphasis on preventing diseases, as well as relieving illness and promoting recuperation or even longevity.

1 Healthcare Theory according to TCM

Historically methods of healthcare originated from the common people, and were later gradually studied and improved by doctors. In turn, doctors guided the common people according to principles of medical science. This process was repeated again and again, with common practice influencing medicine and vice versa.

In China, healthcare incorporates unique modes of thinking that integrate many relevant theories from TCM. These include:
- Four methods of diagnosis (look, listen, ask questions and feel the pulse)
- Eight principal syndromes (yin and yang, exterior and interior, deficiency and excess, heat and cold)
- Five elements (metal, wood, water, fire and earth)
- Five flavors (sour, sweet, bitter, hot and salty)
- Seven emotions (joy, anger, worry, longing, sadness, fear and shock).

There are also other correspondences with internal organs of the body, which are defined differently than they are in Western medicine, and include both the organ and its functional system linked via meridians. While a background in TCM is not necessary to practicing the exercises in this book, it can enhance your experience, and there are many resources available that can help you gain an understanding of TCM's basic concepts.

2 Understanding Meridians and Collaterals

The concept of "meridians and collaterals" may seem mysterious but it is fundamental in TCM. In short, meridians and collaterals are like traffic networks throughout the human body and are special channels for the movement of qi and blood. The main trunk channels are "meridians," while the interrelated branches are "collaterals."

Meridians and collaterals are distributed all over the body, and serve to connect the interior with the exterior, and link the upper and the lower. Together they constitute a system with unique functions, and through mutual communication and influence, they combine the body into an organic whole.

By helping with the circulation of qi and blood, they supply nutrition and promote vital movement within the body. When meridians and collaterals are clear, this promotes the well being of internal organs, whereas blockages bring about the decline and illness of internal organs.

While not a part of Western medicine, the system of meridians and collaterals stems from the accumulation of practice and knowledge over thousands of years, and is a strongly held belief.

Fourteen meridians and collaterals join one another, just like a network of streams and rivers, and circulate qi and blood. First we need to understand what is meant by the positions when referring to meridians and collaterals:

- For the upper limbs, palms (or internal/inner) refer to the inner side of upper limbs while back of the hand (or external/outer) refers to the outer side of the upper limbs. Front refers to parts that are close to the thumbs, while the parts close to the little fingers are referred to as rear.
- The lower limbs are naturally separated into interior, exterior, front and rear parts with the shin bone as the boundary.

For each of the four limbs, there are three different meridian and collateral channels distributed roughly along their two edges and at the center. These twelve, together with Conception Vessel (*ren mai*) and Governing Vessel (*du mai*) about which we will learn more later, jointly constitute fourteen meridians and collaterals:

- Three yin meridians of hands: Running from the internal organs to the hands, the three yin meridians of the hands are distributed along the front, central and rear lines on the inner side (i.e. palms) of the arms.
- Three yang meridians of hands: Running from the hands to the head, the three yang meridians of the hands are distributed along the front, central and rear lines on the outer side (i.e. back of the hands) of the arms.
- Three yin meridians of feet: Running from the feet to the abdomen, the three yin meridians of the feet are distributed along the front, central and rear lines on the inner side of the legs.

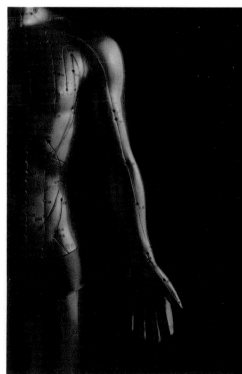

Meridians and collaterals of the human body (image by gettyimages)

- Three yang meridians of feet: Running down to the feet, the three yang meridians of the feet are distributed along the front, central and rear lines on the outer side of the legs.
- Conception Vessel: Originates at the center of the front of the body, inside of the lower abdomen.
- Governing Vessel: Originates below the spine at the center of the rear side of the body.

Yin and yang meridians join one another at the four limbs, yang and yang meridians join one another at the head and face, and yin and yin meridians join one another at the chest and abdomen. They are also interconnected at the Conception Vessel and Governing Vessel.

Acupoints are special areas in the human body through which qi and blood in internal organs and meridians/collaterals are infused and poured out ("point" means "gap" in this case). The points are not isolated on the surface of body. As part of the meridians and collaterals system, these points are closely related to and communicate with tissues and organs deep within the body. Their "communication" is two-way: diseases on the inside are manifested to the outside, while diseases within can be prevented or cured by receiving stimulations from outside. The method for separately tapping meridians and collaterals in Chapter One will provide a detailed introduction to various meridians and collaterals and their important acupoints.

3 Therapies Based on Meridian and Collateral Theory

Meridian and collateral theory lies at the core of the science of acupuncture. Clearing meridians and collaterals through acupuncture can cure different kinds of diseases, as has been shown through experience over many centuries. Modern medical research into acupunctural therapies also indicates that acupuncture can improve the functions of various systems, activate the intrinsic disease

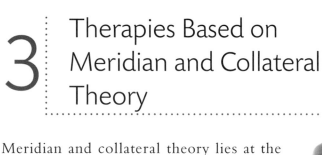

Acupunctural therapy

resistance of the body, and help prevent and treat diseases.

Regrettably it can be somewhat difficult to incorporate acupunctural therapies into healthcare in daily life. Firstly, they must be practiced by professionals. Moreover, the use of needles can often produce special pains and tingling feelings, and will often cause apprehension, or worse, in the patient. Because of this, acupunctural therapies are most effective and accepted when used in conjunction with a specific disease or condition. It is more difficult to use these therapies for regular healthcare and disease prevention, as when no obvious symptoms have appeared, most people would not readily accept them. And they may also not be suitable for treating patients with chronic diseases, as the patients would not endure them over a long time.

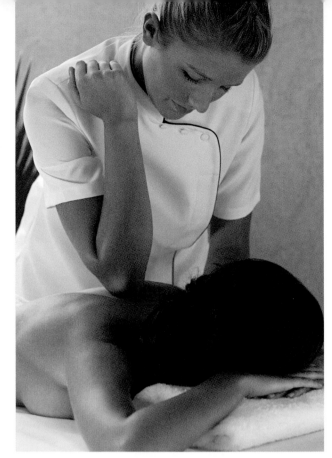

Massaging is a popular therapy for meridian health (image by Quanjing).

Other traditional Chinese therapies, e.g. massage, moxibustion, cupping, scraping and spine-pinching, also take meridian and collateral theory as their theoretical core. While these are popular and widely practiced folk healthcare remedies, they have strong ties to medical treatment.

4 Meridian and Collateral Exercises and Their Curative Effects

I had long been searching for a simple exercise or routine through which practitioners could naturally clear meridians and activate collaterals by stimulating their acupoints, thereby improving health. Unexpectedly, I found what I was looking for quite easily through a chance encounter.

In 1983, during a national academic conference on sports medicine, I was fortunate to encounter Mr. Zhu Heting, a descendant of a Lao Mountain Taoist Priest, who was practicing meridian and collateral exercises. I learned from him this set of exercises, which focuses on the action of tapping acupuncture points. It took about 20 to 30 minutes to practice the set once, after which practitioners would have experienced slight perspiration and would feel relaxed all over.

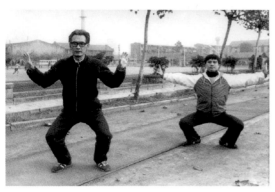

In the 1980s, I learned meridian and collateral exercises from Mr. Zhu Heting.

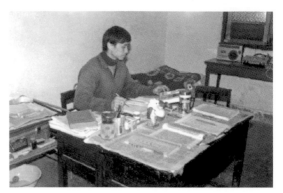

I collected the data of various cardiovascular functions before and after the exercises.

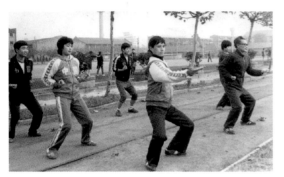

Teaching meridian and collateral exercises with Mr. Zhu

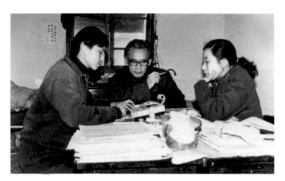

Comparing and discussing the results together with Mr. Zhu

With the help of Mr. Zhu, I ran tests to study the change of various cardiovascular functions before and after the exercises. As it turned out, after practicing the exercises, the pumping force of cardiac muscles and the elasticity of blood vessels increased; the viscosity of blood declined; and the micro-circulation was improved. Not long after teaching these exercises to me, Mr. Zhu visited various parts of China by invitation, and later disappeared into thin air.

In the years since I have been furthering my understanding, innovating and perfecting meridian and collateral exercises while practicing them, as well as incorporating the achievements of others in this field, I have also successively added and developed some actions of clearing and activating meridians and collaterals that are widely used among common folk, e.g. teeth-clicking, ear-drum beating and ear-lifting. Through this extensive research and practice, the set patterns of exercises presented in this book have gradually come into being.

I have observed that many people who practice morning exercises also pat their limbs spontaneously. Regrettably, while patting their limbs, most of these people do not consider the location of their meridians and collaterals, let alone their acupuncture points. They pat their limbs too randomly and apply non-standard techniques with either too much or too little force. Therefore, the beneficial effects will naturally fall far below expectation. However if they knew a bit more about meridians and collaterals and acupuncture points, as well as appropriate techniques, it could make a real difference to their health. Therefore, I felt compelled to provide this book as a resource based on my 28-year practice of meridian and collateral healthcare exercises.

Based on my dedicated practice, this set of exercises has been obviously beneficial to my own energy and spirit, as well as my immunity from illness. These exercises stimulate acupuncture points or meridian and collateral channels through such techniques as pinching, rubbing, clearing, scraping and tapping, which according to TCM, helps clear all of the body's meridians and collaterals, regulate the balance between yin and yang and between qi and blood, invigorate the body, and strengthen its resistance to pathogenic factors. In terms of Western medicine, meridian and collateral exercises can regulate the functions of internal organs, improve cardiovascular function, adjust blood pressure, and increase heat energy consumption.

Many types of people will benefit from practicing these exercises. They can serve as a kind of supplementary therapy for patients with chronic diseases, reinforcing the body and stabilizing or relieving symptoms of hypertension, diabetes and coronary heart disease among other illnesses. The exercises are also suitable for sub-healthy people as well as healthy people who need to maintain and strengthen their body systems and prevent diseases.

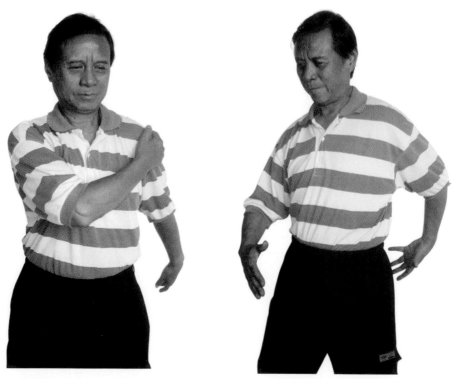

Acquiring knowledge about meridians and collaterals and acupuncture points increases the effect of tapping considerably.

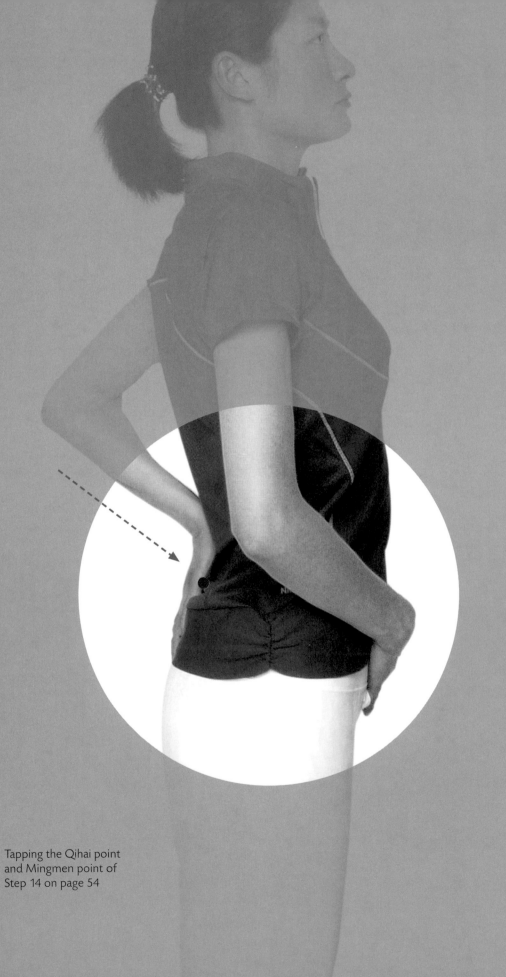

Tapping the Qihai point
and Mingmen point of
Step 14 on page 54

CHAPTER ONE
Methods for Tapping Meridians and Collaterals

The tapping methods introduced in this chapter are relatively simple: The whole body is tapped following a certain sequence and route, using a palm or a simple instrument only. This method clears meridians and collaterals of the whole body, strengthens the body's resistance, and regulates functions of the internal organs. Healthy people will benefit from these healthcare methods as will sub-healthy people and patients with chronic diseases, and the whole-body approach can even prolong life.

For easy mastery, these methods are introduced in three steps from the easiest to the most difficult:

- Tapping areas of the body: While this method does not follow the route of meridian and collateral circulation and intersection, health benefits will arise with devoted practice.
- Tapping the fourteen meridians and collaterals: This method involves a specific sequence and direction of tapping each meridian or collateral, and requires knowledge of the main acupoints.
- Tapping the whole body according to meridians: After acquiring a clear understanding of the fourteen meridians and collaterals, you can pat them in turn according to the sequence of their circulation.

1 Tools for Tapping

Using the palm is the most convenient for tapping meridians and collaterals. The flexibility, width and pliability of the palm make it the most suitable, and you can also fully stimulate the acupuncture points of your palm to reinforce the beneficial effect on health. However it can be difficult for elderly people or those without good flexibility to tap their meridians and collaterals with their palms, especially those in the back and shoulder. Even if they can reach those meridians and collaterals with their palms, they cannot pat them forcefully, thus reducing the effect of tapping.

Some gadgets can be purchased for tapping acupuncture points, e.g. a rubber ball with a handle or a small wooden mallet. Although these gadgets can produce some positive effect, it is difficult to control the tapping force because of their small contact area for tapping and their light weight. This may lead to tapping acupuncture points too violently or hitting bones, causing discomfort. On the other hand, if the points are tapped too weakly or inaccurately, the effect would be undesirable.

The best solution is to produce your own exclusive gadget for effectively tapping your meridians and collaterals (see below 6 steps). Similar to a palm, it has a larger contact area, a certain weight and a pliable patting surface, which ensures comfort and effectiveness while tapping. This gadget can also be used after engaging in sports or physical labor to tap and relax muscles over your whole body.

Since tapping with the palms has many advantages, you can use palms in most cases, and use the above-mentioned gadget to tap only the parts you cannot reach with your palms.

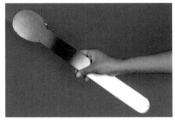

1 Find a five-ply wood board and cut it into an oval shape with a long handle.

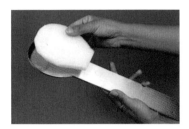

2 Find an oval magnet or other solid material smaller than the oval of the wood board and weighing about 100 to 200 grams. Bind it with adhesive tape or medical tape.

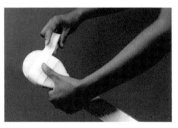

3 Wrap both sides of the five-ply wood board with foam or other cushioning material, using relatively thick cushioning on the sides of the oval section.

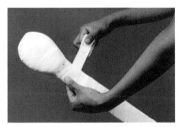

4 Wrap the wood board with adhesive tape or medical tape from top to bottom.

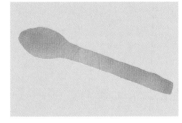

5 The production of your tapping gadget is complete.

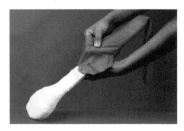

6 Create a fabric coat for the tapping gadget.

2 Tapping Areas of the Body

It is very easy to remember the four areas using this basic method: upper limbs, lower limbs, chest and abdomen, and waist and back. These parts should be tapped according to a certain direction and sequence, as described below.

Although this method is slightly inferior to the other two methods, daily practice brings real health benefits. It can balance yin and yang, and qi and blood, and can strengthen resistance and help prevent disease.

Upper Limbs

Each arm has six meridians and collaterals, which can be roughly regarded as circulating from the shoulder, three going to the palm and three to the back of hand. On each side, the three run to the thumb, middle finger and little finger respectively, and meet at the root of the fingernails.

The inside of the arm contains yin meridians which circulate from top to bottom (shoulder to hand), while the outer side contains yang meridians circulating from bottom to top. Therefore one must follow this circulation when tapping, patting all the yin meridians from top to bottom, and all the yang meridians from bottom to top. Moreover, the inner arm should be patted first. Remember that the front refers to the thumb-side while the rear refers to the side of the little finger (the pinky).

Sequence: interior front line→exterior front line→interior rear line→exterior rear line→interior central line→exterior central line.

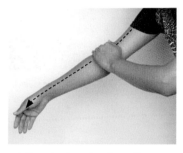

1 Tap the interior front line from top to bottom, from the palm-side shoulder (inside of the shoulder) downward to the inner side of the thumb, along the line of the thumb.

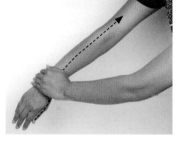

2 Then tap the exterior front line from bottom to top. To do so, you should turn over the hand, and tap upward to the shoulder along the outer (thumb) side, which is now facing downward.

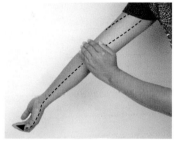

3 Next turn your hand over again to tap the interior rear line from top to bottom. This means from the shoulder downward to the outer side of the little finger along the line of the little finger.

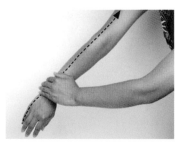

4 To tap the exterior rear line, turn over the hand, and tap upward (from the hand to the shoulder) along the outer side of the little finger.

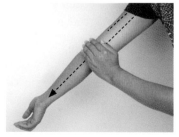

5 The line to follow is the interior central line, in the middle of the inner arm. First tap the interior central line from top to bottom along the line of the middle finger, concluding along the inner side of middle finger.

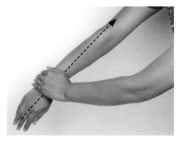

6 Finally tap the exterior central line from bottom to top working your way upward from the outer side of the middle finger to the shoulder.

Lower Limbs

The right and left legs also have six lines respectively. However the directions of the flow of these meridians and collaterals are somewhat different from those of the arms. They can be regarded as circulating from the top part of the thigh to the ankle along three almost parallel lines.

On the outer side of the leg, the outer ankle contains yang meridians which circulate from top to bottom. On the inner leg, the inner ankle contains yin meridians which circulate from bottom to top. They meet one another on both sides of the base of toenails.

While tapping the outer sides of legs, tap all meridians and collaterals from top to bottom, and for the inner legs, you should tap all meridians and collaterals from bottom to top. Moreover the outer sides should be tapped first. This is different from the sequence for tapping the arms. The tapping process for the legs is exactly opposite to that shown above for the arms:

- First tap the exterior front line from top to bottom, from the outer side of the upper thigh downward to the front of the outer ankle.
- Then move to the interior front line from bottom to top. Start at the front of the inner ankle and tap upward to the inner side of the upper thigh.
- Next tap the exterior rear line from top to bottom. Start from the outer side of the upper thigh downward to the rear of the outer ankle.
- Tap the interior rear line from bottom to top, from the rear of the inner ankle upward to the inner side of the upper thigh.
- Then tap the exterior central line from top to bottom. Tap from the outer side of the upper thigh downward to the center of outer ankle.
- Finally tap the interior central line from bottom to top. Start at the center of the inner ankle upward to the inner side of the upper thigh.

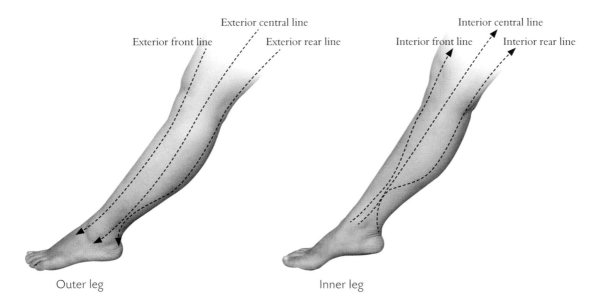

Exterior central line
Exterior front line   Exterior rear line

Interior central line
Interior front line   Interior rear line

Outer leg   Inner leg

Chest, Abdomen and Back

There are three meridians and collaterals on the left and right of the chest and abdomen respectively. From the horizontal midline of the groin, the moving routes can be roughly delineated as being from the exterior to the interior. The exterior and the interior should be gently tapped in turn, from bottom to top.

The Governing Vessel and Conception Vessel should be tapped from bottom to top along the front and rear central lines of the body.

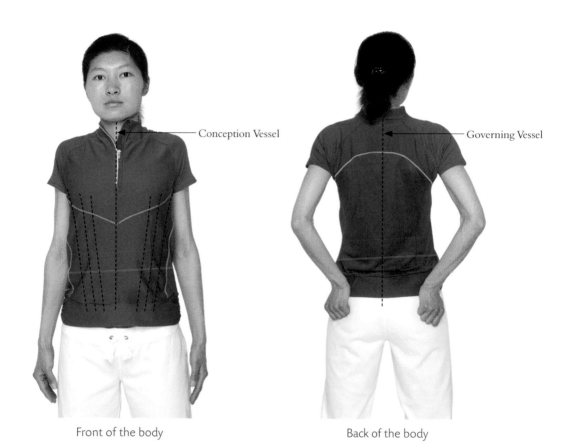

Conception Vessel

Governing Vessel

Front of the body   Back of the body

Head, Face and Feet

The head and face are where yang meridians join one another, and cannot be tapped. The acupuncture points of the head and face should instead be pushed and rubbed strongly and completely until they become hot.

Likewise, as the confluence point of meridians and collaterals, the feet can also be rubbed thoroughly until they become hot. You should wash your foot before tapping, so it may be most convenient to undertake this activity after bathing in the evening or whenever else you may bathe.

3 Tapping the Fourteen Meridians and Collaterals

After mastering the basic practice, you can go on to acquire more knowledge about meridians and collaterals and acupuncture points, and proceed to the following tapping method.

Generally speaking, the qi and blood of twelve meridians and collaterals (excluding for a moment the Conception Vessel and Governing Vessel) circulate continuously, without beginning and end, and without sequence. Then why, when we talk about the circulation and interrelation of these twelve channels, do we start from the Taiyin Lung Meridian of Hand? This is because the lung governs qi all over the body, and qi is the commander of blood, taking the initiative to push blood forward. The smooth flow of qi and blood symbolizes endless life.

Please refer to Meridian Database in Appendices for more information on the location of each acupoint.

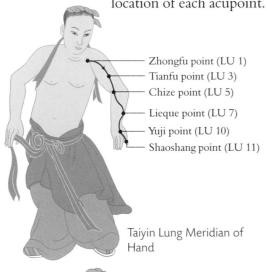

Zhongfu point (LU 1)
Tianfu point (LU 3)
Chize point (LU 5)
Lieque point (LU 7)
Yuji point (LU 10)
Shaoshang point (LU 11)

Taiyin Lung Meridian of Hand

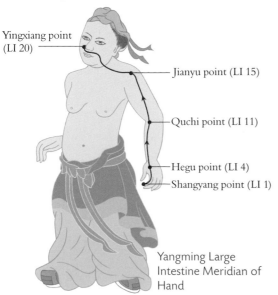

Yingxiang point (LI 20)

Jianyu point (LI 15)

Quchi point (LI 11)

Hegu point (LI 4)
Shangyang point (LI 1)

Yangming Large Intestine Meridian of Hand

Taiyin Lung Meridian of Hand

You will tap sequentially along the interior front line of the arm. Start from the Zhongfu point on the exterior upper side of the front chest, downward to the Shaoshang point of the thumb, moving along the interior front line of the arm in the direction of the thenar eminence, the fleshy mass near the base of the thumb. In this process, the following acupoints, among others, should be tapped: Tianfu point, Chize point, Lieque point and Yuji point.

Yangming Large Intestine Meridian of Hand

Start from the exterior front line of the arm. Tap points one by one starting from the Shangyang point on the fingernail side of the index finger, passing the Hegu point, and continuing upward to the clavicular fossa of the shoulder. Although this sequence ends at the Yingxiang point, do not tap any longer with your palm because the point is located in the face. However it can be tapped gently with a finger. In this process, be sure to tap the following acupoints among others: Hegu point, Quchi point and Jianyu point.

Yangming Stomach Meridian of Foot

The Yangming Stomach Meridian of Foot meets the Yangming Large Intestine Meridian of Hand at the rear of the Yingxiang point. It has a complicated route of circulation.

Although the meridian starts on the body surface at the Chengqi point, like all meridians and collaterals of the head and face, we use the method of pushing and rubbing for acupoints on the head and face. Then you can tap from the outer side of the chest and abdomen downward, across the groin, along the exterior front line of the thigh and calf, downward to the second toe. In this process, the following acupoints, among others should be tapped: Rugen point, Tianshu point, Futu point, Liangqiu point, Dubi point, Zusanli point and Fenglong point.

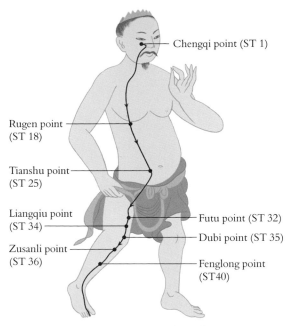

Chengqi point (ST 1)

Rugen point (ST 18)

Tianshu point (ST 25)

Liangqiu point (ST 34)

Zusanli point (ST 36)

Futu point (ST 32)

Dubi point (ST 35)

Fenglong point (ST40)

Yangming Stomach Meridian of Foot

Taiyin Spleen Meridian of Foot

This tapping sequence begins from the inner side of the hallux toe (big toe), upward along the interior front line of the thigh and calf, across the groin, along the outer side of the abdomen, and then to the Dabao point of the midaxiliary line. In this process the following acupoints, among others, should be tapped: Sanyinjiao point, Yinlingquan point, Xuehai point and Jimen point.

Shaoyin Heart Meridian of Hand

Start tapping from the Jiquan point at the center of armpit. Continue along the interior rear line of the upper limbs to the Shaochong point on the inner side of the tip of the little finger. In this process the Shenmen point, among others, should be tapped.

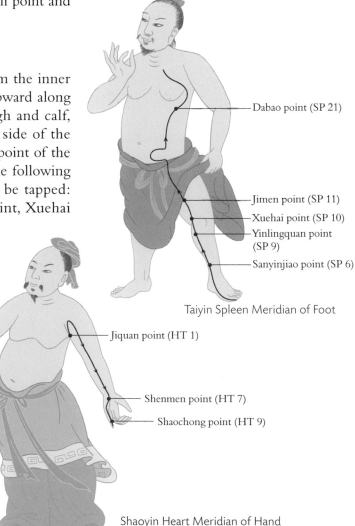

Dabao point (SP 21)

Jimen point (SP 11)

Xuehai point (SP 10)

Yinlingquan point (SP 9)

Sanyinjiao point (SP 6)

Taiyin Spleen Meridian of Foot

Jiquan point (HT 1)

Shenmen point (HT 7)

Shaochong point (HT 9)

Shaoyin Heart Meridian of Hand

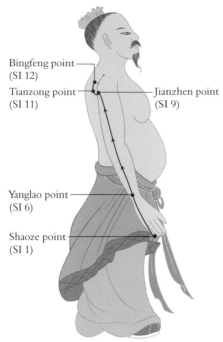

Bingfeng point
(SI 12)

Tianzong point
(SI 11)

Jianzhen point
(SI 9)

Yanglao point
(SI 6)

Shaoze point
(SI 1)

Taiyang Small Intestine Meridian of Hand

Taiyang Small Intestine Meridian of Hand

Please tap from the Shaoze point on the outer tip of the little finger upward along the exterior rear line of the arm, then around the shoulder blade, and finally to the Bingfeng point of the shoulder. In this process the following acupoints, among others, should be tapped: Yanglao point, Jianzhen point and Tianzong point.

Taiyang Bladder Meridian of Foot

Among all meridians, the Taiyang Bladder Meridian of Foot has the largest number of acupuncture points (altogether 134 points). Starting from the Jingming point, it extends from the head through the trunk to the feet, encompassing very complicated branches and moving directions. It passes through the buttocks, continues downward along the exterior rear line of the lower limbs, and finally ends at the Zhiyin point on the exterior edge of the corner of the little toe's nail.

Since this meridian is directly related to the meridians and collaterals of internal organs, it can be used to cure the largest number of diseases. Acupuncture points of the Taiyang Bladder Meridian of Foot are often selected for clinically treating diseases of the urogenital, nervous, respiratory, circulatory and digestive systems. Therefore this route is a vital one for meridian-based tapping, and it can be tapped more often.

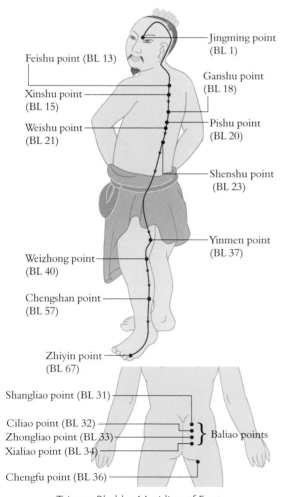

Feishu point (BL 13)

Jingming point
(BL 1)

Xinshu point
(BL 15)

Ganshu point
(BL 18)

Weishu point
(BL 21)

Pishu point
(BL 20)

Shenshu point
(BL 23)

Yinmen point
(BL 37)

Weizhong point
(BL 40)

Chengshan point
(BL 57)

Zhiyin point
(BL 67)

Shangliao point (BL 31)

Ciliao point (BL 32)
Zhongliao point (BL 33)   } Baliao points
Xialiao point (BL 34)

Chengfu point (BL 36)

Taiyang Bladder Meridian of Foot

Tap only from the back, downward along both sides of the spine, across the buttocks, and then further downward along the exterior rear line of the lower limbs. Continue around the rear of the exterior ankle, and finally to the Zhiyin point on the exterior edge of the little toe. In this process, the following acupoints, among others, should be tapped: Feishu point, Xinshu point, Ganshu point, Pishu point, Weishu point, Shenshu point, Baliao points, Chengfu point, Yinmen point, Weizhong point and Chengshan point.

Shaoyin Kidney Meridian of Foot

This tapping sequence starts at the Yongquan point at the center of the sole, continues across the rear of the inner ankle, all the way upward along the interior rear line of the lower limbs. It then moves along both sides of the central line of abdomen, namely only a half cun away from the Conception Vessel. Tapping then continues upward to the Shufu point on the lower edge of the clavicle (collarbone).

Since this Kidney Meridian is chiefly used to cure diseases of the urogenital and endocrine systems, it needs to be tapped often to prevent the hypofunction and premature aging of various internal organs.

While tapping the abdomen, please apply gentle force, being sure not to tap too strongly. In this process the following acupoints, among others, should be tapped: Taixi point, Zhubin point, Dahe point, Qixue point and Shufu point.

Jueyin Pericardium Meridian of Hand

Tap from the Tianchi point in the armpit, along the interior central line of the upper limbs all the way to the Zhongchong point in the tip of the middle finger. In this process, the following points, among others, should be tapped: Tianquan point, Quze point, Jianshi point, Neiguan point, Daling point and Laogong point.

Shaoyang Sanjiao Meridian of Hand

This sequence starts from the Guanchong point. It then continues across the exterior central line of the upper limbs, all the way upward along the rear of the upper arm, to the rear of the shoulder, and then to the Dazhui point. In this process the following points, among others, should be tapped: Waiguan point, Zhigou point, Tianjing point and Jianliao point.

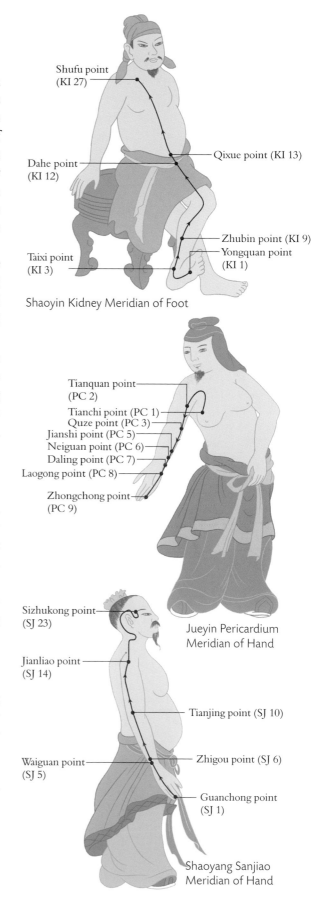

Shaoyin Kidney Meridian of Foot

Jueyin Pericardium Meridian of Hand

Shaoyang Sanjiao Meridian of Hand

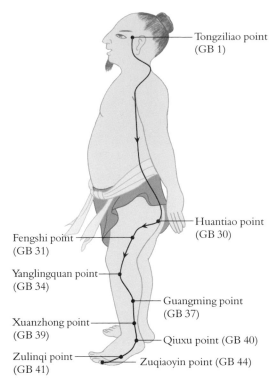

Tongziliao point (GB 1)

Huantiao point (GB 30)

Fengshi point (GB 31)

Yanglingquan point (GB 34)

Guangming point (GB 37)

Xuanzhong point (GB 39)

Qiuxu point (GB 40)

Zulinqi point (GB 41)

Zuqiaoyin point (GB 44)

Shaoyang Gallbladder Meridian of Foot

Shaoyang Gallbladder Meridian of Foot

Start from the Tongziliao point about one centimeter outside the eye, moving from head to foot. The route of circulatory flow and infusion is very complicated. It goes across the Huantiao point, along the exterior central line of the lower limbs, and finally to the Zuqiaoyin point on the exterior edge of the fourth toe.

You can push and rub acupoints of this meridian in the face and head, and there are additional points inside the body that cannot be tapped. Therefore tapping begins only from the Huantiao point on the outer side of buttocks, downward along the exterior central line of the lower limbs, across the front of the exterior ankle and the exterior of the back of the foot, and all the way to the end of the fourth toe. In this process the following acupoints, among others, should be tapped: Fengshi point, Yanglingquan point, Guangming point, Xuanzhong point, Qiuxu point and Zulinqi point.

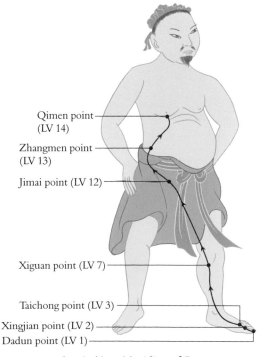

Qimen point (LV 14)

Zhangmen point (LV 13)

Jimai point (LV 12)

Xiguan point (LV 7)

Taichong point (LV 3)

Xingjian point (LV 2)

Dadun point (LV 1)

Jueyin Liver Meridian of Foot

Jueyin Liver Meridian of Foot

Please tap from the Dadun point on the exterior edge of the base of the nail of the hallux toe, along the back of the foot and across the front of inner ankle. Continue along the interior central line of the lower limbs, upward to the groin, then in the direction of the nipple, and to Qimen point. In this process the following acupoints, among others, should be tapped: Xingjian point, Taichong point, Xiguan point, Jimai point and Zhangmen point.

Conception Vessel

The flow of the Conception Vessel is from bottom to top. Located at the center of the chest and abdomen, it starts at the Huiyin point and ends at the Chengjiang point at the mentolabial sulcus of the face (between the chin and lower lip). It governs all of the body's yin meridians, leading to its name. Moving alone in the abdomen and connected with the yin meridians of the whole body, it is also known as "the sea of yin meridians."

Start tapping from the lower abdomen upward along the central line all the way to the Tiantu point at the center of the suprasternal fossa, the small indentation at the top of the breastbone. Since there are many internal organs on this route, please tap gently. The tapping sequence passes through such acupuncture points as the Zhongji point, Guanyuan point, Qihai point, Shenque point, Zhongwan point, Shangwan point and Danzhong point.

Governing Vessel

All of the body's six yang meridians meet at the Governing Vessel, located at the Dazhui point below the seventh cervical vertebra. Due to this convergence, it is also known as "the sea of yang meridians." It governs the qi and blood of the yang meridians of the whole body, and administers reproductive functions.

The Governing Vessel starts at the Baozhong point (including the elixir field and lower energizer [located below the navel], liver, gallbladder, kidney and bladder), and goes out of the Huiyin point, continuing upward to the top of the head along the center of spine, and ending at the Yinjiao point at the connection between the lip frenum and the upper gum.

In this sequence some acupoints cannot be reached for tapping. Please tap only from the tailbone, upward along the central line of the spine, then all the way to the Fengfu point. Since all the acupoints are below spine fissures, they should be tapped heavily with a stronger force. In this process the following acupuncture points, among others, should be tapped: Changqiang point, Mingmen point, Dazhui point, and Yamen point.

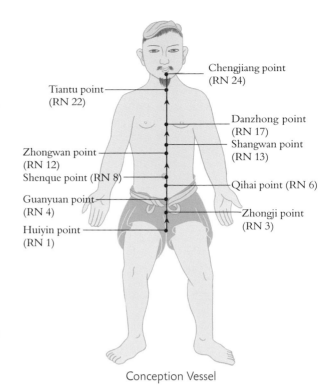

Conception Vessel

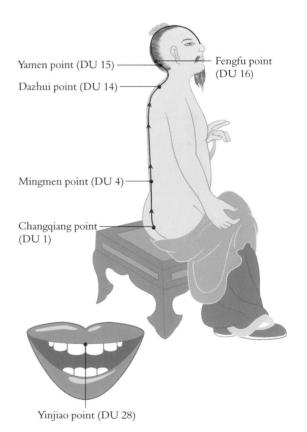

Governing Vessel

4 | Tapping Meridians and Collaterals over the Entire Body

In addition to the methods given above for separately tapping the fourteen meridians and collaterals, you can follow the roadmap below to tap meridians and collaterals of the whole body according to their circulatory flow and infusion.

Please tap them one by one according to the moving flow of these main routes (refer back to instruction in the Section 3 regarding the direction). It is unnecessary to accurately pat each specific acupoint on the meridians and collaterals. First tap the meridians and collaterals of the upper and lower limbs, Conception Vessel and Governing Vessel on one side of the body, then repeat this process on the other side. Finally rub acupoints on the head and face. In this way you are able to tap meridians and collaterals of the whole body.

Roadmap for Tapping Meridians and Collaterals of the Whole Body

Parts	Front Line	Central Line	Rear Line
Interior of Upper Limbs	★Taiyin Lung Meridian of Hand	Jueyin Pericardium Meridian of Hand	Shaoyin Heart Meridian of Hand
Exterior of Upper Limbs	Yangming Large Intestine Meridian of Hand	Shaoyang Sanjiao Meridian of Hand	Taiyang Small Intestine Meridian of Hand
Exterior of Lower Limbs	Yangming Stomach Meridian of Foot	Shaoyang Gallbladder Meridian of Foot	Taiyang Bladder Meridian of Foot
Interior of Lower Limbs	Taiyin Spleen Meridian of Foot	Jueyin Liver Meridian of Foot	Shaoyin Kidney Meridian of Foot

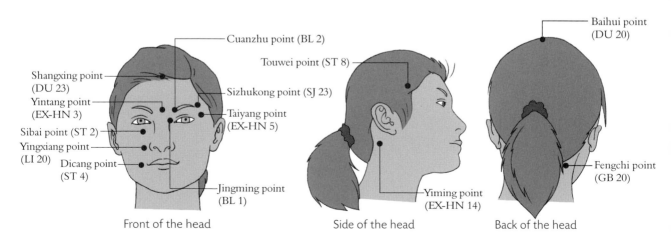

Front of the head — Shangxing point (DU 23), Yintang point (EX-HN 3), Sibai point (ST 2), Yingxiang point (LI 20), Dicang point (ST 4), Cuanzhu point (BL 2), Sizhukong point (SJ 23), Taiyang point (EX-HN 5), Jingming point (BL 1)

Side of the head — Touwei point (ST 8), Yiming point (EX-HN 14)

Back of the head — Baihui point (DU 20), Fengchi point (GB 20)

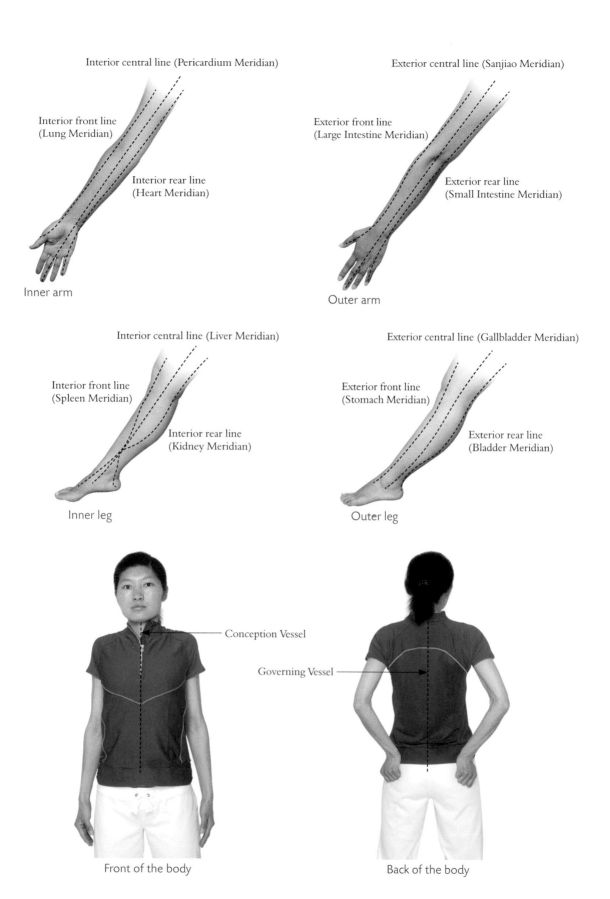

Interior central line (Pericardium Meridian)

Interior front line
(Lung Meridian)

Interior rear line
(Heart Meridian)

Inner arm

Exterior central line (Sanjiao Meridian)

Exterior front line
(Large Intestine Meridian)

Exterior rear line
(Small Intestine Meridian)

Outer arm

Interior central line (Liver Meridian)

Interior front line
(Spleen Meridian)

Interior rear line
(Kidney Meridian)

Inner leg

Exterior central line (Gallbladder Meridian)

Exterior front line
(Stomach Meridian)

Exterior rear line
(Bladder Meridian)

Outer leg

Conception Vessel

Governing Vessel

Front of the body

Back of the body

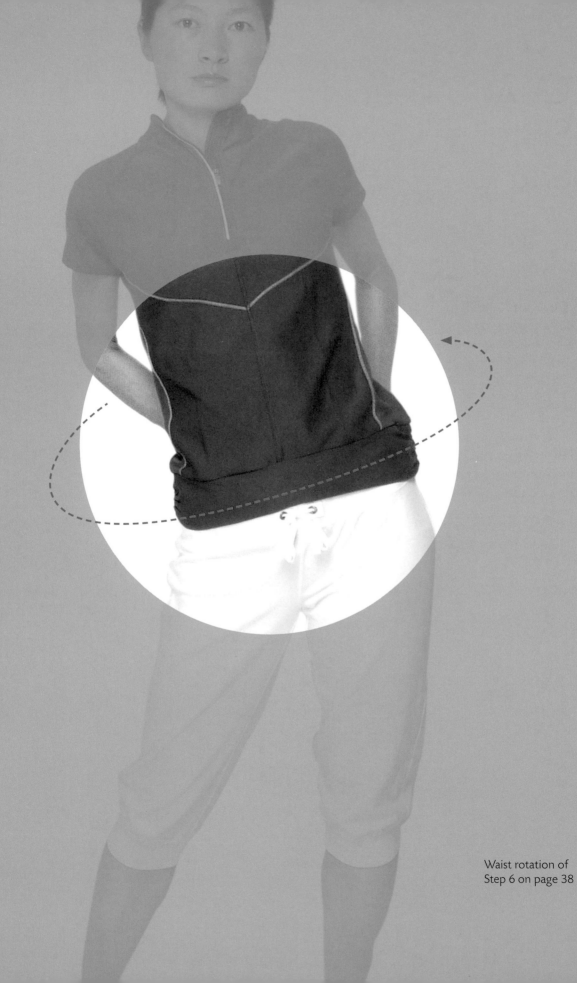

Waist rotation of
Step 6 on page 38

CHAPTER TWO
Sixteen Meridian and Collateral Exercises

In undertaking these exercises please note that each should be practiced according to an 8-beat rhythm. If, for example, the description notes "four 8-beats" that means you should count from one to eight, and then repeat another three times (for a total of four times). Nearly all of the following exercises begin from the "commencing posture."

The practice of the meridian and collateral healthcare exercises is very much dependent on the individual practitioner. Each step can be practiced for a longer or shorter time, and in particular, some targeted actions can be practiced for a longer time. You will gradually find what is most suitable for your own practice, in connection with the contents of Chapter Three, Chapter Four and Chapter Five of this book and according to your own experience, leading to an optimal result.

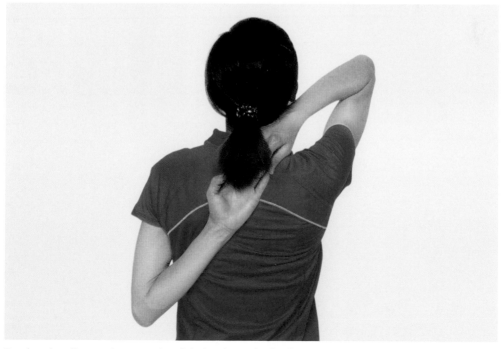

Bend at the elbows, clasp your hands behind your back of Step 10

Step **1** ┊ # Commencing Posture

Efficacy: Mitigating tension in the muscles of the waist and back, and relaxing the spine. It can not only clear meridians and collaterals in the trunk, head and face, but also regulate and relax the mind so that practitioners can more quickly commence their skill practice.

Action: Separate your feet naturally to shoulder-width. Stretch your chest and contract your abdomen. Protrude your hip slightly forward, and with a bit of a knee bend. Imagine that the midpoint of the perineum is exactly opposite the midpoint of the line connecting the Yongquan points of the arches of the feet. Close your eyes and maintain this posture for one to two minutes, breathing calmly.

Note: During the practice, lightly touch your upper palate with the tip of your tongue, relax the muscles of your neck, smile, keep your facial muscles in a slack state, and keep a natural stance of your feet.

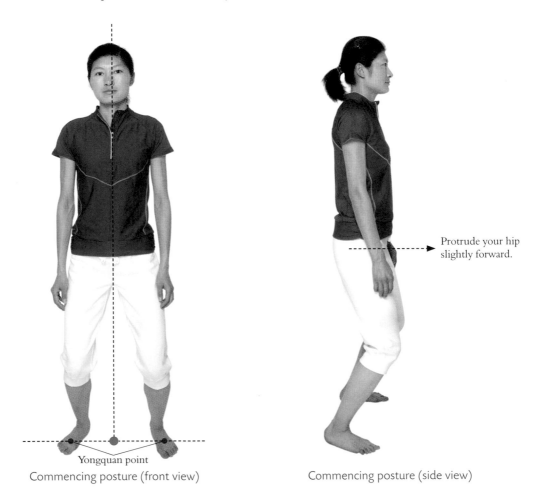

Protrude your hip slightly forward.

Yongquan point

Commencing posture (front view)   Commencing posture (side view)

Step 2 Holding a "Ball" in a Horse-Riding Stance

Efficacy: Clearing meridians and collaterals of the whole body during this gentle and slow circle-drawing movement.

Action: Starting from the commencing posture in Step 1, move your right leg so that you have a wider stance. According to your own tolerance, bend your knee joint into a 90°–135° stance, as if you were riding a horse. Stretch both arms forward, naturally separate your fingers, and position your arms as if you are holding a large ball in your arms. Maintain this arm position, as you move from the waist, hip, shoulder and back to make full circles in different directions (left, right, top and bottom). Repeat the action for four 8-beats.

Note:

1. During the practice be sure to slightly rotate your neck along with your action, and move your eyes to follow the direction of the "ball." This allows you to gradually bring unity to the movement, concept and spirit.

2. This practice can be used as a warm-up for other meridian and collateral exercises. It can also be practiced separately in your spare time, or when you are in a bad mood, to relax the whole body. In particular, by practicing this action, office workers who sit a lot or have frequent eye strain can relieve their physical and mental fatigue.

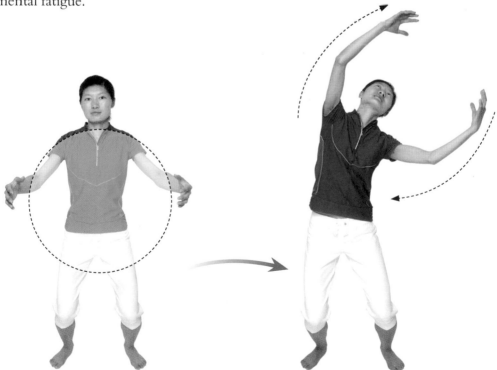

Hold a "ball" in a horse-riding stance.   Make a circle from left to right.

Step 3 Hand-Throwing and Tiptoeing

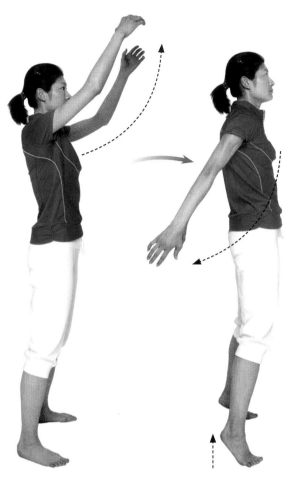

Efficacy: Using all the large muscle groups of the upper and lower limbs, coordinated with deep breathing, this step can strengthen the activity of your qi and blood. It can also link up your meridians and collaterals, and in particular it can make the operation of qi and blood at the end of your limbs and trunk smoother.

Action: Starting at the commencing posture, throw both your hands forward above your head, and breathe deeply at the same time. Next, try to throw both your hands from the front of your chest backward along the sides of your body, lifting both heels and exhaling. Repeat the action for two to four 8-beats.

Note: It is very important to adjust your breath to coordinate with the action.

Throw both your hands forward above your head.

Stand on tiptoe and throw both your hands backward.

For Whom Is This Action Most Suitable?

Currently the comprehensive treatment of chronic diseases includes low-intensity and long-duration movement of large muscle groups. This can help increase the pumping force of the cardiac muscle, increase returned blood volume, dilate peripheral vessels, improve micro-circulation, increase heat consumption, enhance the balance and coordination of body, and increase the muscle strength of the upper and lower limbs.

Therefore, this movement can produce a desirable auxiliary effect in stabilizing or mitigating the symptoms of such chronic diseases as hypertension, diabetes and mild coronary heart disease.

Step 4 : Pressing and Releasing

Efficacy: Long-term practice of these actions can improve the functions of internal organs and mitigate such symptoms as tinnitus, headache, dizziness, insomnia, hypomnesis (poor memory), forgetfulness and mental decline.

Action:

1. Press both auricles (outer ears) with the centers of your palms, fingers facing toward the back of the head. Massage as if drawing a circle from the rear to the front; repeat this process five times.

2. Tightly press both your auricles. Rapidly and strongly flip your head back three times with intercrossed index fingers and middle fingers; you may hear a sound like "bang-bang."

3. Next, practice the action of pressing and releasing with your palms in turn. The last round of pressing should last for a longer time and should be practiced more strongly. Then open both your palms rapidly, and you can hear a buzz.

Note: This action enables your ear canal to repeatedly and suddenly change from an airtight state to an open state, producing a rapid change of air pressure. The conduction of sound and the change of air pressure can improve the blood circulation of the inner ear and help with hearing.

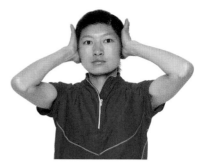

Massage your auricles.

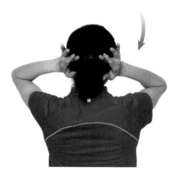

Flip your head back.

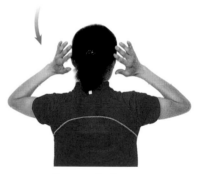

Press and release.

Auricular Therapy

Your auricles, or outer ears, are covered with many points (known as otopoints) that are interconnected with internal organs, the four limbs and the entire skeleton. Otopoints are deeply linked with various physiological or pathological changes of the body. Therefore auricular therapy, or otopoint massaging, is used in TCM for therapy and health maintenance.

The action above is a modification of ear-drum beating, an effective healthcare method that has been in practice among common folk for a long time, with the addition of the actions of massaging the auricles and pressing and releasing with your palms in turn. This allows the otopoints to be mechanically massaged, and the inner ear is massaged as well with a change of pressure, thus enhancing the effect of the traditional ear-drum beating practice.

Step 5 | Teeth-Clicking and Swallowing

Efficacy: Practicing this action often can improve blood circulation at the tooth root and gum, and can considerably help to secure teeth. In addition it will increase the secretion of saliva, which contains substances that help promote digestion. Therefore this action is very helpful for maintaining normal functions of the spleen and stomach.

Action: Gently click together the upper and lower teeth; repeat this process 20 to 100 times; stir with your tongue the saliva accumulated in your mouth and then slowly allow it to enter your digestive tract.

Step 6 | Rotating Various Parts of the Body

This action involves your eyes, neck, shoulders, waist, hips, knees and ankles. The amplitude of rotation for each part should increase gradually, and the rotation continue slowly, clockwise and counterclockwise in turn. By changing direction, the rotation stops at intervals, enabling qi and blood to run through your whole body.

Eye Rotation

Efficacy: The circulation of qi and blood is accelerated through movement of the eye muscles, thus relieving eye-fatigue and improving eyesight.

Action: Try to open both eyes to look forward levelly, preferably at a tree or other focal point in the distance. Stay like this for eight beats. Keeping your head and body motionless, rotate both your eyes. First slowly rotate your eyes in the following order: left→top→right→bottom→left. Gradually increase the amplitude of rotation. After rotating your eyes clockwise and counterclockwise in turn for eight beats (eight circles), stop and close your eyes to rest for eight beats. Then repeat the above-mentioned process.

Neck Rotation

Efficacy: The circulation of qi and blood is accelerated through movement of the neck muscles, and rotation allows for neck muscles to be slowly pulled, thus relieving neck-muscle fatigue and helping to prevent and cure cervical degeneration.

Action: Maintain the commencing posture, with both your hands naturally slack at your sides and your body motionless. Begin to slowly rotate your neck for eight circles in the following order: left→rear→right→front→left. Increase the amplitude of rotation gradually. At the end of this process, stretch your head and hands backward, staying motionless for eight beats. Then repeat this process in the opposite direction. At the end stretch your head and hands backward again, staying motionless for eight beats.

Note: Those who already suffer from cervical degeneration with dizziness due to nerve pressure are advised to turn the neck only slightly. They should stop at once if there is discomfort in the course of turning the neck.

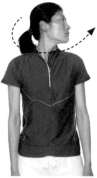

Rotate your neck.

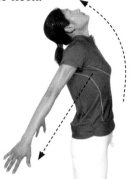

Stretch backward.

Shoulder Rotation

Efficacy: This action can fully activate and pull muscles of the shoulder and neck, clear meridians and collaterals of the shoulder and neck, and prevent and cure cervical degeneration and periarthritis of the shoulder.

Action: Maintain the commencing posture, with both your palms lying naturally on the exterior of your thighs. Your palms will slide up and down as you slowly shrug and rotate your shoulder for eight circles in the following order: up→forward→down→back→up. At the end of this process keep your hands motionless on the exterior of your thigh, and forcefully stretch your chest and head forward with your eyes gazing at the sky. Maintain this posture for eight beats. Repeat the above-mentioned process in an opposite direction. End with both your hands again motionless on the exterior of your thigh, your chest and head forward, and eyes upward, holding the posture for eight beats.

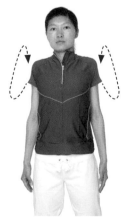

Shrug and rotate your shoulders.

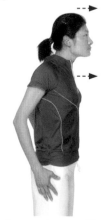

Stretch your chest and head forward.

Waist Rotation

Efficacy: This action can fully activate and stretch muscles and ligaments in the lumbosacral region, and massage and clear meridians and collaterals in this region. It has a positive effect on preventing and curing chronic lumbocrural (lower back) pain, e.g. strain of the lumbar muscles.

Action: Separate your legs to shoulder-width, and slowly rotate your waist clockwise and counterclockwise for two 8-beats (circles) in turn. While rotating your waist always keep your hands on your waist with clenched fists. Support both sides of the spine in the lumbosacral region, or any uncomfortable region, with your metacarpal phalangeal joints (the first knuckle, at the base of the finger), so that the rotary force produced by twisting at the waist results in a massaging action from the metacarpal phalangeal joints.

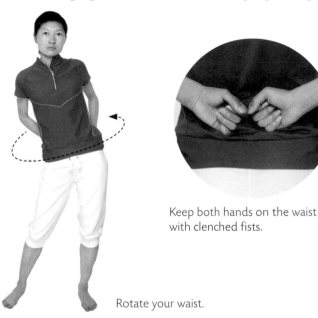

Keep both hands on the waist with clenched fists.

Rotate your waist.

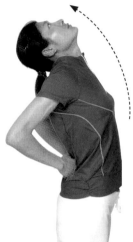

Support waist with both fists, with waist moving forward and neck stretching backward.

Hip Rotation

Efficacy: This action can fully activate and stretch the muscles and ligaments of the perineum and hip, and produce a beneficial effect on the functions of the urogenital system.

Action: Separate your legs to shoulder-width, slightly bending your knees. Place both hands on your hips, and rotate your groin clockwise and counterclockwise in turn. During the rotation, continuously lift up from the bottom of your groin at the same time. Try to keep the parts above your waist still and upright, only rotating from the groin area. Rotate two 8-beats (circles) in each direction.

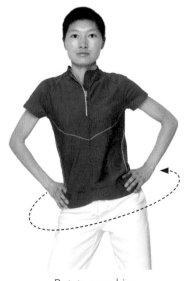

Rotate your hip.

Knee and Ankle Rotation

Efficacy: Engaging the knee and ankle joints and the muscles of the legs, this action helps to clear meridians and collaterals of the lower limbs and enhance flexibility of the joints. It can be used as an auxiliary practice to prevent and cure joint pain.

Action: Separate your legs so that they are as broad as your shoulders. Slightly bend your knees, gently pressing them with your palms. Simultaneously rotate your knee joints in the same direction, then rotate in the opposite direction. Rotate in each direction for two 8-beats (circles). Next rotate your ankle joints in each direction for two 8-beats. End by straightening your legs and pressing your knees with your palms.

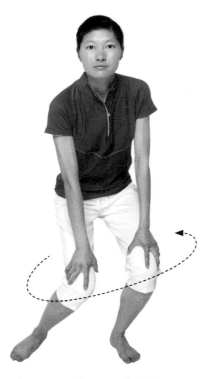

Rotate your knees and ankles.

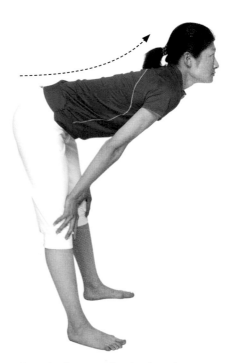

Press both your palms backward; straighten your knees.

Step 7 : Pinching and Rubbing

Efficacy: This action can clear meridians and collaterals in your head, and produce some adjuvant therapeutic effect for such common symptoms as headache, dizziness, insomnia, forgetfulness and decrease of mental capacity/acuity.

Action:

1. Place the fingertips of both your hands horizontally along the line of eyebrows, spreading outward as far as the temples. Gently pinch and rub the following acupuncture points for four 8-beats: Yintang, Cuanzhu, Sizhukong and Taiyang, etc.

2. Now gradually push your fingertips upward, remaining in a straight horizontal line, from the forehead to the top of the head, then progressing to the occiput (back of head). Gently pinch and rub each part with your ten fingertips at the same time. After four 8-beats, stop when your fingertips have reached the line of the Shangxing point and Touwei point (near the hairline), and gently pinch and rub them for four 8-beats.

3. Continue to pinch/rub and push upward. After four 8-beats, stop again when your fingertips have reached the line of the Baihui point (at the top of the head), and gently pinch and rub the point for four 8-beats.

4. Continue to pinch/rub and push upward to occiput. After four 8-beats, when your fingertips have reached the Fengchi point below the occiput, forcefully pinch and rub the Fengchi point. This should be for four 8-beats, however you should only use your thumbs.

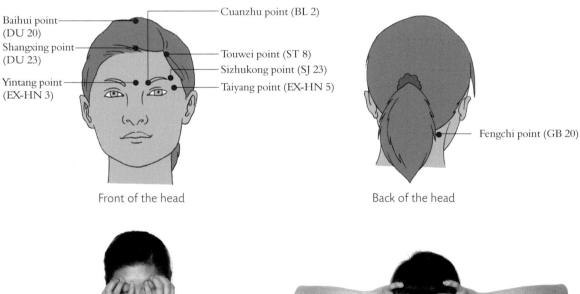

Baihui point (DU 20)
Shangxing point (DU 23)
Yintang point (EX-HN 3)
Cuanzhu point (BL 2)
Touwei point (ST 8)
Sizhukong point (SJ 23)
Taiyang point (EX-HN 5)
Fengchi point (GB 20)

Front of the head   Back of the head

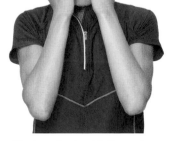

Pinch and rub with fingertips.

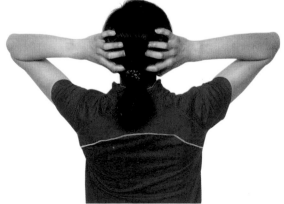

Rub the Fengchi point with both thumbs.

Step 8 | Combing and Scraping

Efficacy: This action can help nurture your hair, improve your eyesight and relive headaches caused by some chronic diseases. It also provides a way to refresh yourself and restore your consciousness.

Action: Slightly separate the fingers of both hands. Comb your hair from the front to the rear for four 8-beats one to two times. You should use your fingers and palms for combing and scraping at the same time, and intentionally let your fingers cross such acupuncture points as Yintang, Touwei, Shangxing, Baihui and Fengchi. When you comb downward from the top of your head, use the hypothenar (the little finger side of your palm) instead to apply clamping force from the palms to scrape from the rear of ears all the way to the neck. The acupuncture points scraped in the meantime include Yiming and Fengchi.

Note: After combing and scraping, your head and neck will feel a sense of heating, which denotes that your qi and blood are running smoothly. The many meridians and collaterals that meet at your head and neck are connected with one another, thus adding blood supply to your head and neck.

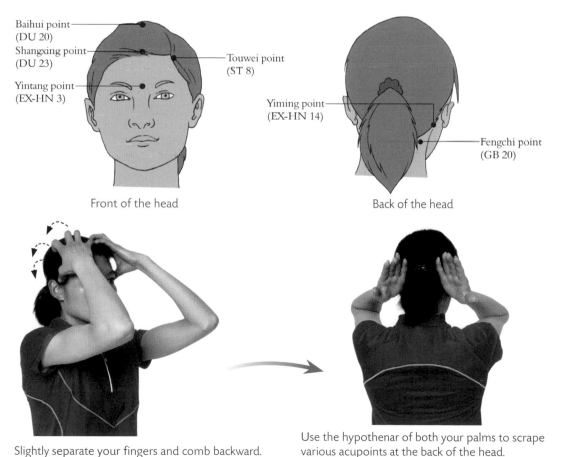

Baihui point (DU 20)
Shangxing point (DU 23)
Yintang point (EX-HN 3)
Touwei point (ST 8)

Yiming point (EX-HN 14)
Fengchi point (GB 20)

Front of the head

Back of the head

Slightly separate your fingers and comb backward.

Use the hypothenar of both your palms to scrape various acupoints at the back of the head.

Pushing and Rubbing

This step uses the hands to push and rub. Using these actions on your face and chest/abdomen can clear meridians and collaterals in these areas, nourish your five sense organs, and strengthen the functions of various systems.

Push and Rub Your Face

Efficacy: This action can improve the qi and blood operation in the entire face, nourish and regulate your five sense organs, improve your complexion, and reinforce the disease resistance of your upper respiratory tract.

Action:

1. Horizontally push and rub your forehead. Comb your face by pushing and rubbing with the pads of both middle fingers. Push and press from the inner edges of eyebrows to the temples for two 8-beats.

2. Still using the pads of both middle fingers, push and rub your eye sockets by drawing circles in opposite directions (i.e. both from interior to exterior at the same time) along your orbit, for two 8-beats respectively.

3. Push and rub your face up and down. Move in the following order: ophryon (the midpoint of the forehead just above the top of the nose)→hair line→eye socket →sides of nose→corner of mouth→ophryon. In this process you should intentionally apply force to such acupuncture points as Yintang, Jingming, Sibai, Yingxiang and Dicang. When your middle fingers are used for pushing and rubbing, your thumbs should always push and

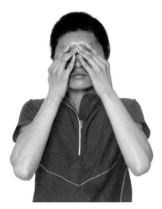

Horizontally push and rub your forehead.

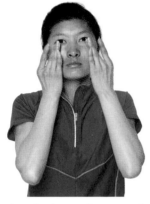

Push and rub your face up and down; apply force to the Sibai point.

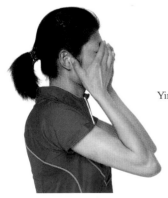

Push and rub your face up and down (side view).

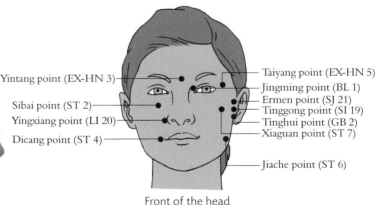

Yintang point (EX-HN 3)
Sibai point (ST 2)
Yingxiang point (LI 20)
Dicang point (ST 4)

Taiyang point (EX-HN 5)
Jingming point (BL 1)
Ermen point (SJ 21)
Tinggong point (SI 19)
Tinghui point (GB 2)
Xiaguan point (ST 7)

Jiache point (ST 6)

Front of the head

rub back and forth along the outer side of your face, i.e. along the line of the Xiaguan point in front of the ears, the Ermen point, Tinggong point and Tinghui point as well the Jiache point and other points. Other fingers should be used naturally to press other parts of your face, and should produce force along with upward and downward pushing and rubbing. Two 8-beats are acceptable.

Push and Rub Your Chest and Abdomen

Efficacy: This action can improve the functions of the cardiovascular, respiratory, digestive and urogenital systems.

Action: Using a bit of force, push, rub and press with both your palms along the central line of your chest and abdomen by continuously drawing circles toward the left and the right and from top to bottom for four 8-beat. When both palms are upward, inhale; when both palms are downward, exhale. This will allow acupuncture points in your chest/abdomen to be massaged in an all-round way.

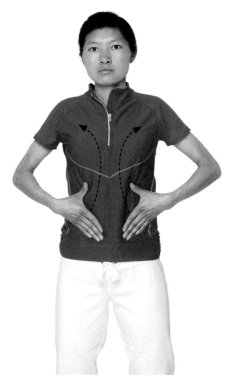

Inhale when both palms are upward.

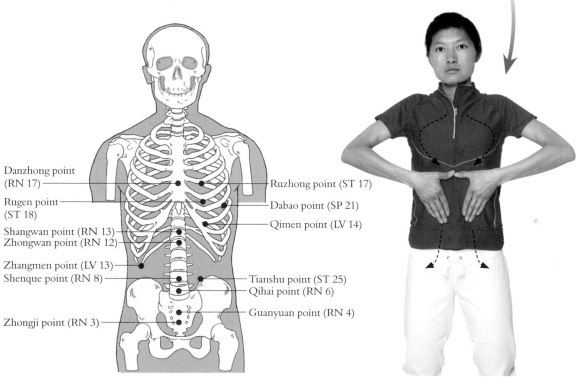

Danzhong point (RN 17)

Rugen point (ST 18)

Shangwan point (RN 13)
Zhongwan point (RN 12)

Zhangmen point (LV 13)
Shenque point (RN 8)

Zhongji point (RN 3)

Ruzhong point (ST 17)

Dabao point (SP 21)

Qimen point (LV 14)

Tianshu point (ST 25)
Qihai point (RN 6)

Guanyuan point (RN 4)

Front of the body

Exhale when both palms are downward.

Step 10 Pulling and Pushing

When you apply the force of pulling and pushing to certain points, you stimulate different muscles and enhance the flexibility of joints, which can relax tendons and activate collaterals. With continued practice, the effect will be more obvious, especially in respect to tonifying the kidneys and maintaining the health of the neck and shoulder.

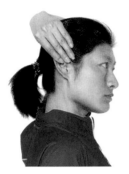

Ear-lifting

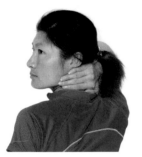

With your right hand held horizontally, pull your neck and rotate your head to the left.

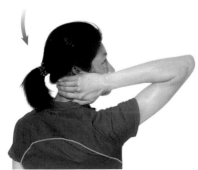

Pull your neck and rotate your head rightward.

Ear-Lifting

Efficacy: This action can tonify the kidney, strengthen your physique, and improve resistance to senility. It is also effective in curing irregular menstruation and, in men, nocturnal emission and impotence.

Action: Stretch one of your arms across the top of your head, holding the ear on the opposite side. Slowly lift and pull your upper ear. As you are applying continuous force, suddenly relax your hand. Do this for two 8-beats for each side.

Note: According to TCM, the ear is the external aperture of the kidney, which governs the bones and marrow. During the action of ear-lifting, the part of the ear that you hold is the fossa triangularis, an area corresponding to the body's endocrine and reproduction functions.

Horizontal Neck Pulling

Efficacy: Preventing and curing cervical degeneration.

Action: Turn your head to the left, placing your right hand behind your neck from the right side reaching from the back of the neck to the lower jaw. Tightly pinch your neck with your entire palm. Then pull it backward with a gentle force, and at the same time slowly rotate your head to the right for two 8-beats. Use your left hand to repeat this action in the opposite direction for two 8-beats.

Note: As this practice causes your neck muscles to be pressed and pulled horizontally, it affects the neck's blood circulation. This can help to soften and dissipate pathological changes caused by arthritis, etc., including obstructions of the qi and blood of the neck, stiffness of the shoulder and neck, fasciitis and fascia nodules. Therefore this practice is beneficial in the prevention and curing of cervical issues.

Shaking Your Hands behind Your Back

Efficacy: This action can clear your meridians and collaterals and activate your qi and blood. It helps to prevent and cure cervical degeneration, periarthritis of the shoulder, fasciitis of the shoulder and back, and strain of the waist and back muscles.

Action:

1. Stretch both hands horizontally and shake them behind your back. Pull them backward strongly, lifting at the same time. Draw your abdomen in and move your chest forward, stretching your head backward, and then slowly rotating your head to the left and right. The entire action lasts for four 8-beats.

2. Bend at the elbow with one arm extending above the head and one remaining at your side. Clasp your hands behind your back. Shake the two hands up and down behind your back. While withdrawing your abdomen, stretching your chest forward and your head backward, try to tightly pull the hands with force. Practice the action with your left and right hands in turn; two 8-beats respectively.

Note: This action is particularly recommended to people who sit for long periods or use computers extensively. Every 20 minutes or so, you can practice this step (preferably while standing). Breathe deeply at the same time, which can eliminate your physical and mental fatigue and relieve the above-mentioned chronic diseases and symptoms.

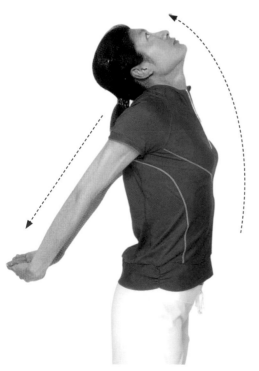

Stretch both your hands horizontally and shake them behind your back.

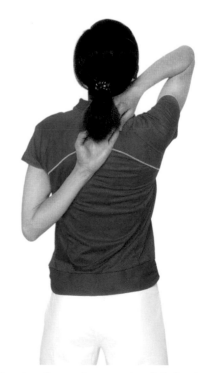

Bend at the elbows, clasp your hands behind your back.

Step 11 Bending and Pressing

Bending and pressing is a common TCM technique. Through its pulling action, this technique can clear meridians and collaterals by stretching joints, muscles, tendons and ligaments. In this way, it not only reinforces qi and blood circulation but also enhances the flexibility and ductility, or pliability, of the body, particularly the limbs.

The ductility of human body depends on that of the joints, and flexible joints are less susceptible to injury. In addition, ductility can help to enhance the coordination and flexibility of your whole body. People with good coordination and flexibility are more resilient during sports, appear steady and outgoing in daily life, have a good bearing, and are more amenable. Therefore frequent practice of the "bending and pressing" step is advisable for preventing and reducing athletic strain as well as for overall well-being.

"Bending and pressing" includes many actions. Several common actions are explained below.

Embrace Your Head and Press Your Elbows and Shoulders

Efficacy: This action lays emphasis on pulling the shoulder joints and muscle groups on the outer side of trunk. It can help to reinforce the pliability of your shoulders and waist, and prevent and cure waist pain and periarthritis of the shoulder.

Action: Raise both your arms above your head. Grasp and press your elbows with the opposite palms, encircling your head. Add pressure to the left and right side respectively. You can add a side-bend of waist at the same time. Practice this action with your left and right hands in turn; two 8-beats respectively.

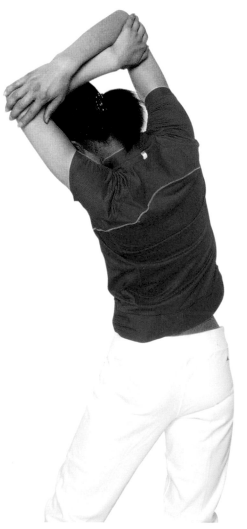

Embrace your head and press your elbows and shoulders.

> **For Whom Is This Practice Not Suitable?**
>
> Hypertensive patients should not attempt this action; it is safer for them to press their legs from a sitting or standing posture.

Stretch Your Arm around Your Neck and Grasp Your Ears

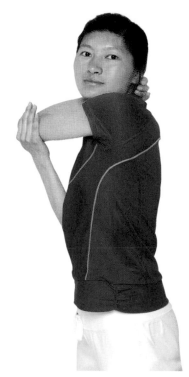

Stretch your arm around your neck and grasp your ear.

Efficacy: This action can help to enhance the pliability of your shoulders and neck muscles, and prevent and cure periarthritis of the shoulder and cervical degeneration.

Action: Bend your upper arm on one side and stretch it around your neck from the front, attempting to grasp your ear (the one the same side as the arm you are stretching). You can use the palm on the other side to press the exterior of your elbow. Twist at the side of your body to increase the pulling effect on your shoulder and neck. Practice this action with your left and right hands in turn; two 8-beats respectively.

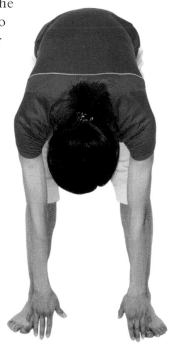

Bend at the waist and touch the ground.

Bend Your Waist and Touch the Ground

Efficacy: This is the most common and widely-used exercise, with the same efficacy as leg-pressing.

Action: Draw both your legs close to each other or separate them so that they are shoulder-width. Bend forward from your waist. Try to touch the ground with both your palms without bending your knees. Draw your face as close to your legs as possible. Make your action rhythmic, practicing it for four 8-beats.

Step 12 : Letting Go and Taking in Breath

Efficacy: By deeply regulating your breath and changing the pressure of your chest and abdomen, as well as the strength of the muscles of your whole body, you can improve the qi and blood operation in your internal organs, nourish your body and achieve health benefits such as reinforcing the functions of your heart and lungs, and promoting heat consumption.

Action:

1. Move from commencing posture to horse-riding (squatting) posture.

2. Inhale deeply. Bend your elbow, semi-clench the fists of both hands with the center of the fists upward, and place your hands at your sides.

3. At the end of a deep inhalation, change your right fist into a sword-pointing posture (i.e. index and middle finger straightened with the other three fingers clenched).

4. Exhale deeply. Then apply invisible force to slowly point toward the front until your upper arm is completely stretched out, horizontal to the ground. This is the part of the move known as "letting go" of your breath.

5. Along with a deep inhalation, hold your breath and apply invisible force to slowly retrieve your right arm. Gradually restore the fist to a semi-clench, placing it back on the side of your body. This is the "taking in your breath" stage.

6. Repeat the above-mentioned process with your left hand. Exercise both sides in turn in this way with the action taking 8 beats. Practice for two 8-beats respectively.

Note: Meridians and collaterals connect the interior with the exterior and the upper and lower parts of body, and it is necessary to maintain a flow of breath. Therefore practitioners cannot suppress their breath during the practice. They must always exhale and inhale deeply and smoothly in turn; otherwise their blood pressure could fluctuate, which is unfavorable especially for hypertensive patients.

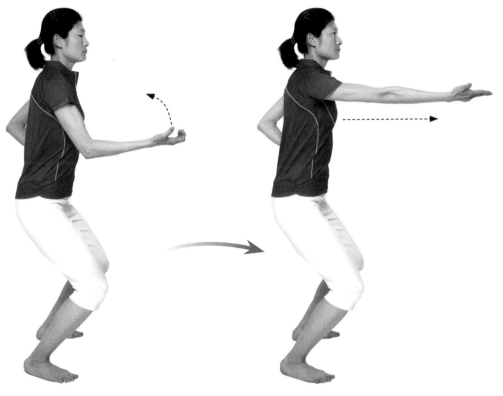

Take in your breath.   Let go of your breath.

Step 13 Pushing a "Wall"

Efficacy: This practice is done in what as known as a squatting and rising posture, with a focus on regulating your breath. This allows you to maintain and strengthen your legs, enhance the coordination and stability of your whole body, promote the flow of peripheral blood back to your heart, and clear the qi and blood in your body.

Note: During the practice, always breathe deeply and do not suppress your breath. Alternate deep exhalations and inhalations, breathing smoothly; otherwise fluctuation of blood pressure may occur, which can be harmful for hypertensive patients. This method of breathing takes a different approach than that of the "letting go and taking in breath" technique, and it is superior in this case because it reinforces the functions of your heart and lungs, and promotes heat consumption.

Action:

Beat 1: Start from the commencing posture. With the center of the palm facing downward, raise both your arms to the side horizontally, and inhale deeply.

Beat 2: Sweep your arms down in an arc, crossing them in the front of your chest. Exhale deeply at the same time.

Beats 3–4: After a deep inhalation, maintain a bend in your elbow and rotate your bent arms so they form a "V" from each shoulder. The center of your palms should face outward. End with a deep inhalation.

Beats 5–6: Slowly push away your arms on both sides toward a horizontal position. Gradually take a squatting position, exhaling deeply at the same time. End your exhalation after coming to a full squat with both arms completely straightened.

Beat 7: Raise both your hands horizontally, and slowly stand upright along with a deep inhalation.

Beat 8: Slowly return your arms to your sides, and exhale deeply. This 8-beat action together comprises the "pushing a wall" exercise in a squatting and rising position. Be sure to complete this sequence fluidly at one stretch, repeating the sequence four times, i.e. four 8-beats.

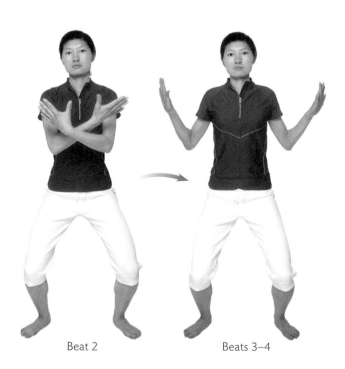

Beat 2

Beats 3–4

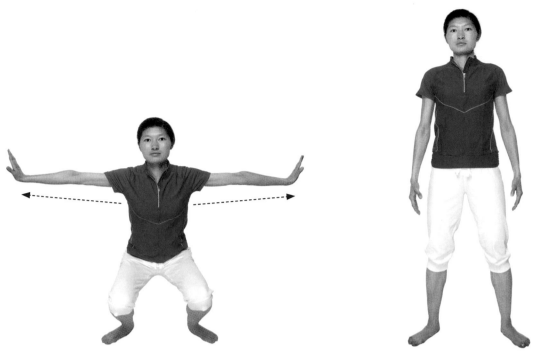

Beats 5–6   Beat 8

Advancing Your Practice

This action requires the support of the legs. Please practice this action carefully and progressively, from easy to difficult steps, taking caution against falling. If you cannot squat fully, you can practice semi-squatting first, building up to a full squat, which will achieve a much better effect.

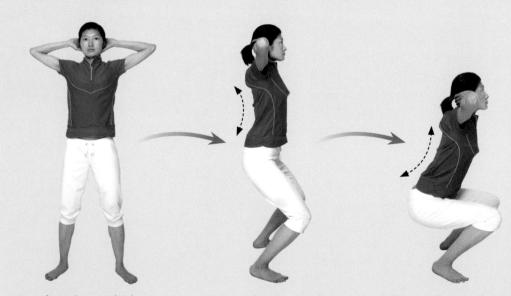

Start from the standard commencing posture. Hold your head with both your hands, elbows pointing out. Straighten at the waist.

Bend your knees to 90 degrees and then stand up. Repeat this 10 to 20 times.

When you feel comfortable, you can do this exercise moving from a deep squat to a standing position. Repeat this process 10 to 20 times.

Step 14 : Tapping the Whole Body

"Tapping the whole body" refers to tapping the main acupoints of your body and the circulating parts of your meridians and collaterals with the palm, back of the hand or different parts of the fist. Of all the methods, this is the most concentrated practice for directly stimulating acupoints, and it is the most important step. While it requires study and knowledge about acupoints it will achieve the best effects on your health.

The main points of the tapping technique are: finding points accurately; applying force skillfully; keeping your qi and blood calm and smooth; and maintaining your breath.

In the tapping process, the interaction between different parts of your hand and the body parts you are tapping can stimulate acupoints on the fourteen meridians and collaterals. Accurately tapping the acupoints or circulating parts of the meridians and collaterals will help to clear the meridians of the whole body.

During the practice you should pay attention to the coordination of breathing. Inhale before tapping, and exhale at the moment when your body is tapped, taking care not to suppress your breath. Proper breathing can not only enhance the effect of clearing qi and blood, but can also prevent the fluctuation of blood pressure that can be caused by breath suppression.

Note:

1. You should begin each tapping process from the commencing posture, and stretch both your arms. After each sequence, you should return to the commencing posture.

2. In the tapping process, you often need to twist your waist to drive the force of your hands. Moreover it is preferable to use force that is strong enough to create an ache in each acupoint or body part.

3. Each of the parts selected for tapping generally needs to be tapped for at least four 8-beats.

4. There are many acupoints and parts that can be tapped in relation to different health conditions. The following focuses on some common parts, and while all these parts can be tapped, you may select to choose only some of them for tapping, based on your own situation.

5. Please note that acupuncture points of head and face should not be tapped. Please choose instead other techniques for clearing, including pinching and rubbing; combing and scraping; and pushing and rubbing.

For Whom Is This Practice Not Suitable?

People with "hemorrhagic physique," e.g. reduction of platelets, vitamin deficiency, subcutaneous hematoma or bruising, and gum bleeding during tooth brushing, must tap their meridians and collaterals gently, or perhaps not practice the tapping technique.

Tapping the Upper Limbs

Efficacy: This action can clear and smooth qi and blood and regulate yin and yang.

Action: Tap with your palm, starting from the front side of your arm moving from top to bottom. Then tap the rear side of arm from bottom to top. Tap each side for 8 beats, evenly distributed, alternating front and rear sides for four 8-beats respectively. When tapping some of the main acupoints, you can use more force and tap them for a longer period, e.g. the Neiguan point on the inner arm, and the Hegu point, Waiguan point and Quchi point on the outer side of the arm.

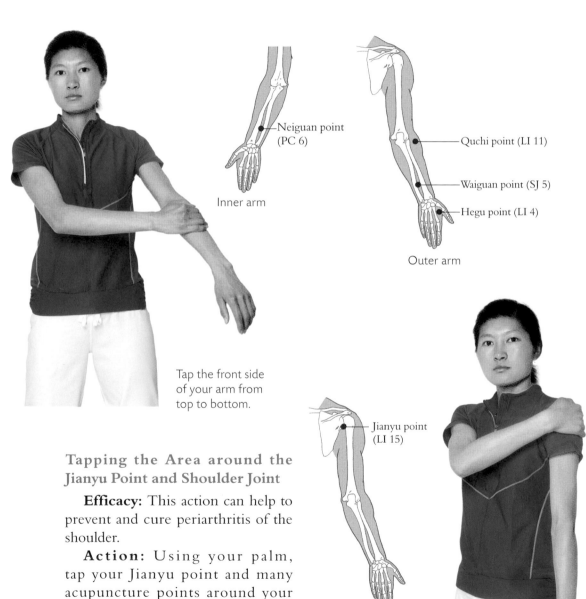

Neiguan point (PC 6)

Inner arm

Quchi point (LI 11)

Waiguan point (SJ 5)

Hegu point (LI 4)

Outer arm

Tap the front side of your arm from top to bottom.

Tapping the Area around the Jianyu Point and Shoulder Joint

Efficacy: This action can help to prevent and cure periarthritis of the shoulder.

Action: Using your palm, tap your Jianyu point and many acupuncture points around your shoulder joint. Tap the left side and right side in turn; two 8-beats respectively.

Jianyu point (LI 15)

Outer arm

Tap your Jianyu point.

Tapping the Feishu Point and Dazhui Point

Efficacy: This action can clear qi movement, and enhance disease resistance of the upper respiratory tract.

Action: Tap with your palm, touching the Feishu point and Dazhui point, which are common points for treating lung diseases and the common cold. Tap the left and right side in turn; two 8-beats respectively.

Tapping the Tianzong Point

Efficacy: This action can treat shoulder and back pain.

Action: Tap with your palm. If you tap the point accurately and forcefully, you will feel tingling in the entire shoulder as well as the back and arms. Tap the left and right side in turn; two 8-beats respectively.

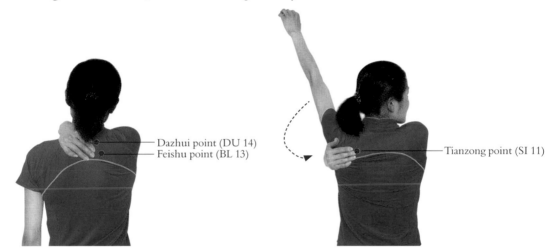

Tap your Feishu point and Dazhui point.

Tap your Tianzong point.

Tapping the Jianjing Point and Bingfeng Point

Efficacy: This action can prevent and cure pain in the region of the shoulder and back, or shoulder and neck.

Action: With your palm, tap the left and right side in turn; two 8-beats respectively.

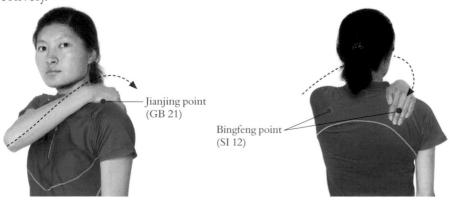

Tap your Jianjing point.

Tap your Bingfeng point.

Tapping the Qihai Point and Mingmen Point

Efficacy: This action can regulate the functions of your digestive, urogenital and endocrine systems.

Action: With your palms opposite each other, tap with both palms at the same time. Tap the center of your abdomen and waist. In addition to tapping the Qihai point and Mingmen point, you should also include the Shenque, Guanyuan, Zhongji and Tianshu points in your abdomen and the Yaoyangguan point in your waist. Tap for four 8-beats.

Note: Be sure to inhale at the moment of each tap. This can not only prevent your internal organs from being damaged but also enhance the effect of relaxing tendons and activating collaterals.

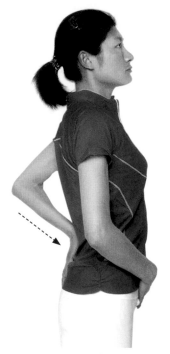

Tap your Qihai point and Mingmen point.

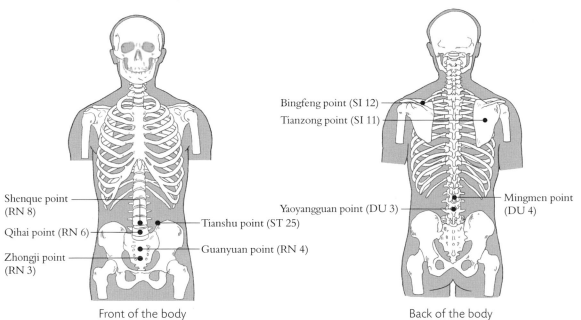

Shenque point (RN 8)

Qihai point (RN 6)

Zhongji point (RN 3)

Tianshu point (ST 25)

Guanyuan point (RN 4)

Front of the body

Bingfeng point (SI 12)

Tianzong point (SI 11)

Yaoyangguan point (DU 3)

Mingmen point (DU 4)

Back of the body

Tapping on and along the Spine

Efficacy: This action can clear and reinforce the yang qi of the whole body, and regulate the functions of internal organs.

Action: With the back of your hand, tap the left and the right side of your back in turn. Tap from your sacrum upward gradually, alternating right and left sides. Tap up to the point where you cannot stretch your hand upward any further. Next, tap downward gradually in turn, slowly back to the sacrum. Repeat this up and down and side to side; tapping four 8-beats is equivalent to one sequence. Repeat this four times, i.e. four sequences each consisting of four 8-beats.

Note: Using the back of your hand and alternating your tapping from right to left helps to give amplitude to the action and increase force. It would be very difficult to do this with your palm. In the process of tapping, twist your waist to help drive both arms, and swing your arms away from the body to use momentum and increase force. At the moment when the body is tapped, your arm should bounce back immediately, to generate a strong explosive force.

It is beneficial to tap to the height of your mid-back, so that you can tap more acupoints. It is difficult for most beginners to manage this, and range of action will come through increased practice and flexibility.

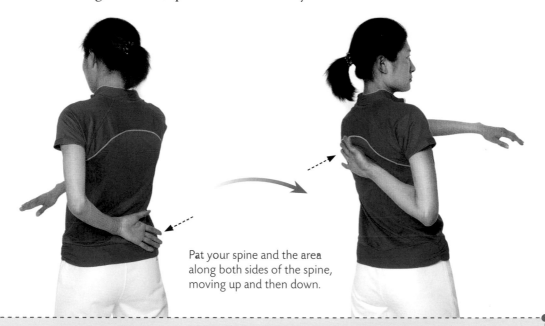

Pat your spine and the area along both sides of the spine, moving up and then down.

Practise This Exercise Separately

"Tapping on and along the spine" can stimulate the Governing Vessel and Taiyang Bladder Meridian of Foot, which are distributed on and along the spine. It can also clear acupoints of all internal organs, completely regulate the functions of various internal organs, and reinforce the primordial yang of the body.

This action requires amplitude, a great deal of dorsal stretching and rotation of the shoulder joint, and coordinates with bending at the waist. Therefore it can also produce the positive effect of preventing and curing periarthritis of the shoulder, lumbar strain, pain of the waist and leg, and cervical degeneration.

This action is especially important among the entire meridian and collateral exercises, and can be practiced separately. It is not only suitable for healthy people but also sub-healthy people who need to enhance their health level. Moreover, for many chronic patients, this action is also effective rehabilitative training.

Practice this action separately one to three times every day. Tap up and down and side to side four times of four 8-beats each time, and you will certainly reap amazing benefits.

Tapping the Buttocks and the Outer Thigh and Calf

Efficacy: This action can prevent and relieve pain in the waist and legs, invigorate the stomach, cleanse the gallbladder and promote urination.

Action: This tapping action uses a clenched fist. You should tap with the palm side of the fist. Tap both sides of your body at the same time. Begin tapping at the Huantiao point (the place where a natural depression forms on the outer side of the gluteus maximus when standing). Be sure you are in the commencing posture, and begin tapping from top to bottom, squatting to reach your calf, and then bending at the waist to finish at the ankle. Move downward, tapping once to twice, working for four 8-beats each time.

Meridians and Collaterals and Acupoints of the Outer Leg

Three yang meridians of the foot are distributed on the outer side of the thigh and calf. The Yangming Stomach Meridian of Foot, Shaoyang Gallbladder Meridian of Foot, and Taiyang Bladder Meridian of Foot are located at the front, center and rear respectively of the outer leg. All of them move from top to bottom.

You should apply more force and spend a longer time when tapping the following acupoints:

- Yangming Stomach Meridian of Foot: Futu point, Liangqiu point, Zusanli point and Fenglong point
- Shaoyang Gallbladder Meridian of Foot: Huantiao point, Fengshi point, Yanglingquan point, Guangming point and Xuanzhong point
- Taiyang Bladder Meridian of Foot: Chengfu point, Yinmen point, Weizhong point and Chengshan point.

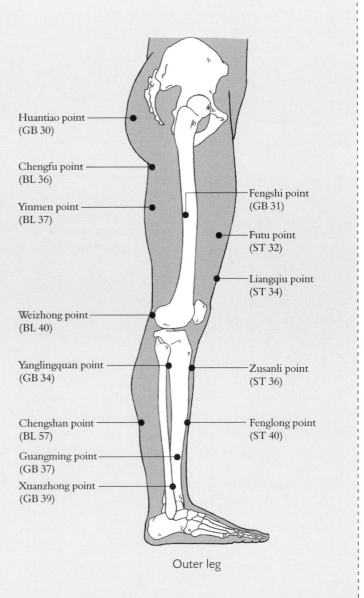

Huantiao point (GB 30)

Chengfu point (BL 36)

Yinmen point (BL 37)

Fengshi point (GB 31)

Futu point (ST 32)

Liangqiu point (ST 34)

Weizhong point (BL 40)

Yanglingquan point (GB 34)

Zusanli point (ST 36)

Chengshan point (BL 57)

Fenglong point (ST 40)

Guangming point (GB 37)

Xuanzhong point (GB 39)

Outer leg

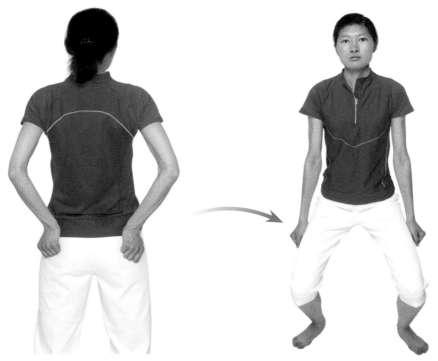

1. Pat the Huantiao point on your hip.

2. Pat your thigh (front view).

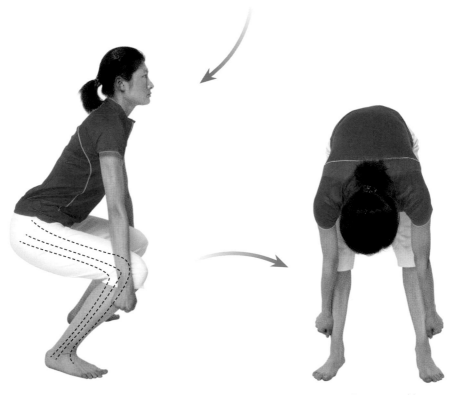

3. Pat your calf (side view).

4. Pat your ankle.

Tapping the Inside of the Thigh and Calf

Efficacy: This action can prevent and release pain of the waist and leg, and invigorate the spleen, liver and kidney.

Action: Clenching your fists, tap both sides at the same time. It is most convenient and comfortable to tap with the hypothenar of your fist. Begin tapping the upper side of the inner ankle, moving from bottom to top. Work in a sequence from front to center to rear. Tap the inner side of calf, and move upward bit by bit, tapping each part once or twice; four 8-beats each time.

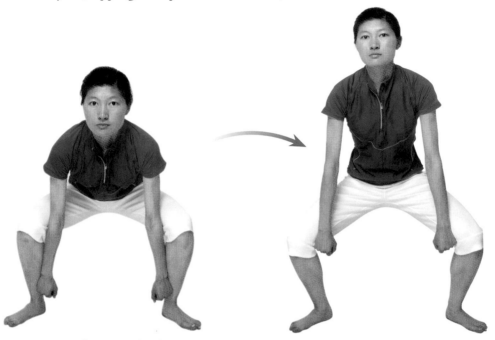

Begin tapping at the inner side of the ankle.   Tap the inner sides of both legs at the same time.

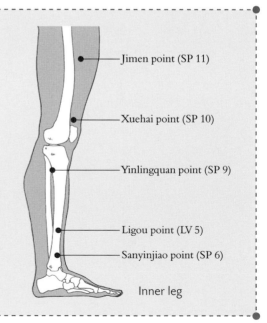

Meridians, Collaterals and Acupuncture Points on the Inner Side of the Leg

On the inner side of the thigh and calf, three yin meridians of the foot are distributed. The Taiyin Spleen Meridian of Foot, Jueyin Liver Meridian of Foot and Shaoyin Kidney Meridian of Foot are located at the front, center and rear respectively. All move from bottom to top.

More force should be applied while passing the following acupoints, which should also be tapped for a longer time: Sanyinjiao point, Ligou point, Yinlingquan point, Xuehai point and Jimen point.

Jimen point (SP 11)

Xuehai point (SP 10)

Yinlingquan point (SP 9)

Ligou point (LV 5)

Sanyinjiao point (SP 6)

Inner leg

Tapping the Abdomen and Chest

Efficacy: This action can bring plentiful vital essence to the whole body, regulate functions of the internal organs, eliminate depression and elevate your mood.

Action: Semi-clench your fist, and tap gently with your palm. In the process of tapping, do not apply the same force as you would to other parts. Make sure to be gentle, otherwise your internal organs may be harmed. In the process of tapping, inhale deeply. Then, with a faster rhythm, move from bottom to top along each of the three routes of movement for the Conception Vessel and three yin meridians of foot. Tap from outside to inside. This can enhance the clearing and smoothing of qi activity. At the same time, utter an "Ah" sound and continuously exhale. In each cycle of exhalation and inhalation, complete tapping from bottom to top once. You should tap the left side of abdomen and chest with your right palm and vice versa.

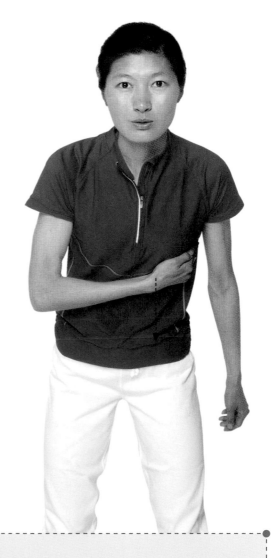

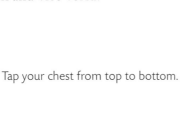

Tap your chest from top to bottom.

Important Centers: Abdomen and Chest

The central line of the abdomen and chest is the moving direction of the Conception Vessel. The three routes arranged on both sides respectively are the moving directions of the yin meridians of the foot. After passing through the groin, the spleen meridian, liver meridian and kidney meridian are arranged from outside to inside. Finally they enter the abdomen and respectively join their corresponding internal organs.

In contrast, all three yin meridians of the hand start from the chest and circulate to the hand. Therefore the abdomen and the chest are important centers where the vital essence of the whole body concentrates. Gentle tapping and deep breathing is beneficial for enhancing vital essence, and regulation of organs and mood.

Step 15 Swaying and Shaking

Efficacy: This action serves to relax your body before completing the set of meridian and collateral exercises. It can further reconcile and clear meridians and collaterals of the whole body. This practice can rapidly ease tension and get rid of your fatigue and other problems. It is very helpful for calming your mind, preventing and curing psychoneurosis and hypertension, and relieving the pain of various joints.

Action: Separate your feet so they are as broad as your shoulders, slightly bend your knees, let your arms droop, separate your fingers naturally and close your eyes. Sway and shake your whole body back and forth and left and right for one to three minutes. In the process, you should remain loose and try to involve all joints of your limbs and trunk, including the neck, shoulder, elbow, wrist, waist, hip, knee and ankle, in this action so as to achieve the effect of full relaxation. The amplitude of swaying and shaking can increase gradually and then decrease gradually; the speed can also follow this pattern, slowly coming to a rest at the end.

Note: Spending several minutes "swaying and shaking" during work breaks will certainly provide myriad benefits to office workers.

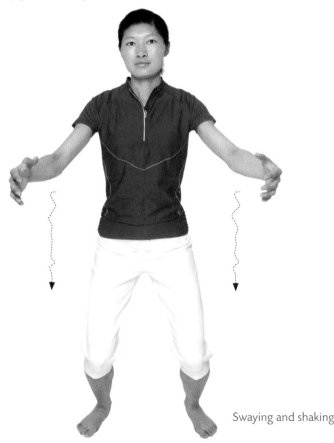

Swaying and shaking

Step 16 Closing Eyes Meditatively

Efficacy: This action can bring considerable relaxation and comfort to your whole body. Furthermore it can smooth your qi and blood, reconcile your yin and yang, refresh your spirit and provide tranquility. This will help you to slowly enter a state of self-oblivion after your practice and allow you to fully enter into a meditative state.

Action: As the last step, Step 16 is the ending posture. After completing the preceding step (swaying and shaking), separate your arms to the left and right, and with palms facing upward. Inhale deeply and raise both arms over your head. Then with palms facing downward, press your arms downward to hug yourself. Exhale at the same time, crossing and overlapping your hands naturally, and placing your palms at the center of your abdomen.

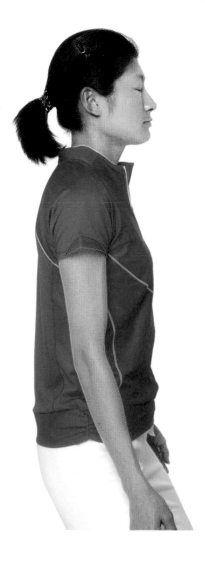

At this stage, your body position and breathing follows the same guidelines as for the commencing posture. Close your eyes and stand still, breathing into the abdomen slowly and gently. Try to concentrate your attention on the ups and downs of your palms and abdomen. Meditate on pleasant things and beautiful scenery you have experienced, and push aside annoying and depressing thoughts. Let your practice come to its end naturally, after two to three minutes or after your eyes open of their own accord. Your meridian and collateral exercises are now at an end, and you should feel quite refreshed, physically and spiritually.

Note: If the last two steps are practiced together one to three times a day (three to five minutes a time), they can have a regulating role for many people with nervous and mental issues.

Ending posture with concentrated attention

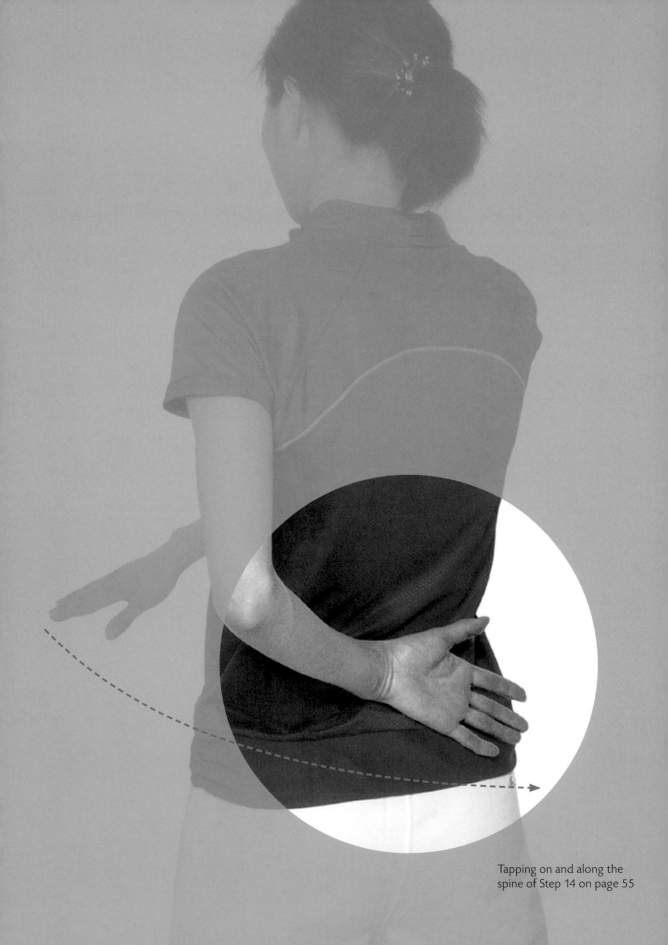

Tapping on and along the
spine of Step 14 on page 55

CHAPTER THREE
Meridian and Collateral Methods for Healthy People

Increasing awareness of health issues and how best to treat and prevent them has many benefits. Not only can it considerably reduce various diseases in individuals and prolong their lives, but it also has a huge social and economic benefit. Therefore, if you are currently healthy, you should be vigilant in learning about and acting to continuously maintain your healthy state.

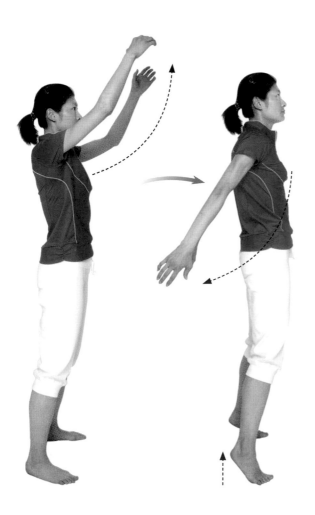

Step 3 hand-throwing and tiptoeing

Meridian and Collateral Exercises

It is best to spend about 20 minutes every day practicing all the sixteen steps of the meridian and collateral exercises described in Chapter Two. You can also choose the following six steps from among these sixteen steps to practice in conjunction or separately. You should develop a habit of practicing them at least once or twice every day.

1. Step 3 hand-throwing and tiptoeing: 100 to 200 times

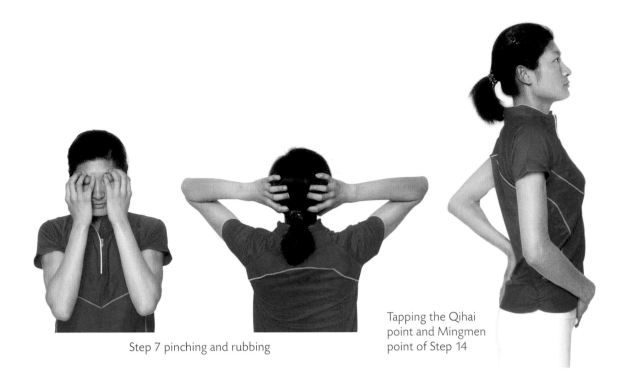

Step 7 pinching and rubbing

Tapping the Qihai point and Mingmen point of Step 14

2. Step 7 pinching and rubbing: four 8-beats

3. Tapping the Qihai point and Mingmen point of Step 14: four 8-beats

4. Tapping on and along the spine of Step 14: tap up and down and side to side four times; four 8-beats each time

5. Step 15 swaying and shaking: 1 to 3 minutes

6. Step 16 closing eyes meditatively: 1 to 3 minutes

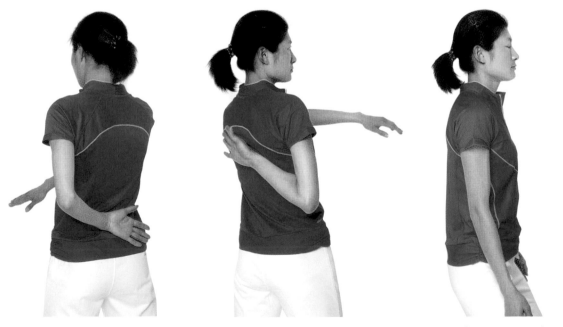

Tapping on and along the spine of Step 14

Step 16 closing eyes meditatively

Self-Massaging

These techniques can help to maintain the functions of your spleen, stomach, liver, kidney and heart.

1. Acupoint pinching and rubbing of the Zusanli, Sanyinjiao and Neiguan points: Each should be gently rubbed for 30 to 60 seconds, once or twice a day.

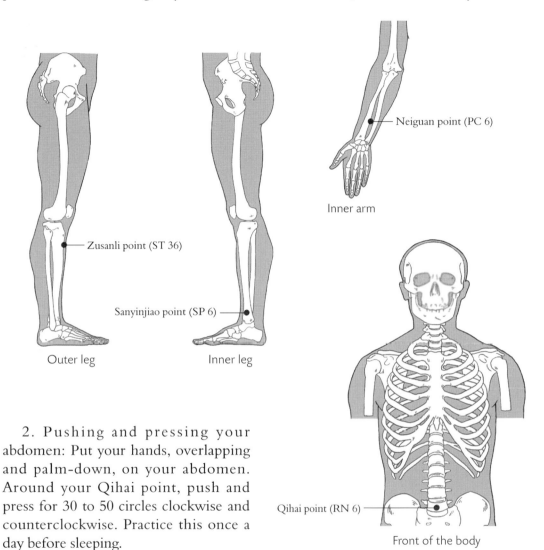

Neiguan point (PC 6)

Inner arm

Zusanli point (ST 36)

Sanyinjiao point (SP 6)

Outer leg   Inner leg

2. Pushing and pressing your abdomen: Put your hands, overlapping and palm-down, on your abdomen. Around your Qihai point, push and press for 30 to 50 circles clockwise and counterclockwise. Practice this once a day before sleeping.

Qihai point (RN 6)

Front of the body

Additional Tips

It is important for healthy people to develop and maintain good life habits. You should be sure to pay attention to proper nutrition, exercise moderately, keep your mind calm and release tension, and refrain from smoking and drinking. In particular, please do not ignore fatigue. However busy you are, you should find time to move about outdoors. Please choose such aerobic exercises as fast walking, jogging, swimming, hiking and dancing, which can not only keep you fit but also regulate your mood, maintaining your physical and mental health.

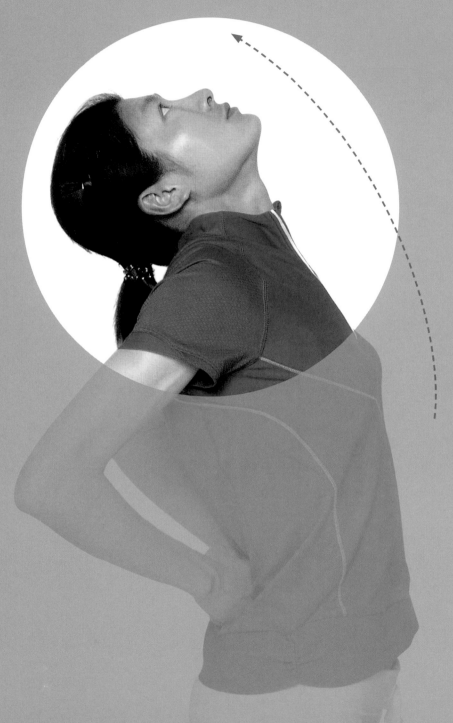

Waist rotation of
Step 6 on page 38

CHAPTER FOUR
Meridian and Collateral Methods for Sub-Healthy People

In modern life we are increasingly confronted with a more hurried pace of work, decreased manual labor and physical activities, and the development of some bad living habits. This can lead the metabolism to become disorderly, the functions of internal organs to weaken, physical agility to decline, or even illness to occur more often.

However due to their own regulation and strong compensation functions, most people tend to be between the states of healthiness and illness in most cases. Although they always feel uncomfortable somewhere, the result of physical examination shows that they are "healthy." This is called "a pre-sick state" in traditional Chinese medicine, and called "the third state" or "over-fatigue syndrome" in modern medicine. We refer to this as a sub-healthy state.

Manifestations of sub-health vary greatly from person to person and include the change of skin, hair and body-shape; the hypofunction of various organs and systems; and the change of sleep, spirit and mental function, among other signs. However these abnormalities are usually nothing but subjective sensations. No organic cause would be found at medical institutions.

According to statistics of WHO (World Health Organization), the sub-healthy population is currently increasing in many countries and regions. In the opinion of many experts, sub-health will become the No.1 killer in the 21st century. By investigating thousands of employees, the Japanese Public Health Research Institute found out that 35% of people had been suffering in a state of sub-health for at least half a year. About six million Americans are suspected to be in sub-healthy states every year.

Although sub-health is not a disease, its further development inevitably brings about diseases. Therefore it is vital to search for the signs of sub-health, and strive to identify and relieve it before it degenerates.

According to the findings from numerous epidemiological surveys, common sub-healthy states closely related to pathological changes include: obesity, hyperlipidemia, insomnia, general malaise, cold hands and feet, visual fatigue, loss of appetite, mental strain, depression, baldness and constipation. This chapter offers some healthcare methods that people in these common physical states can practice themselves to say goodbye to sub-health as soon as possible.

1 Obesity

It is important to first understand the definition and causes of obesity, and evaluate your own situation. Then you can develop a corresponding plan to control and reduce the fat in your body.

Obesity is related to such factors as heredity; disorders of nerve, mental and endocrine regulation; problems with metabolism; eating too much and/or the wrong type of food; and decreased physical activity. In general, obesity can be classified into the following two types according to whether there are underlying endocrine-metabolic diseases:

Simple obesity: This is caused by the proliferation and/or hypertrophy of some fat cells in the human body. In one case, this can be attributed mainly to heredity, and then to over-nutrition. This kind of obesity is also called "constitutional obesity," and for this type it is ineffective to only control the diet. The other case is caused mainly by over-nutrition, next to heredity. In people with this form, fat cells are simply hypertrophic but not proliferous, and obesity can be controlled through diet. Therefore, this kind of obesity is called "acquired obesity." To increase health and weight loss, people with this kind of obesity benefit from physical exercise.

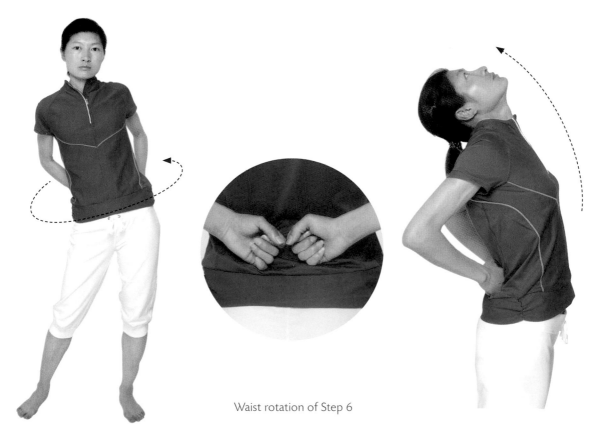

Waist rotation of Step 6

Secondary obesity: People with this kind of obesity have endocrine-metabolic diseases, e.g. hypofunction of the hypothalamus, pituitary gland, thyroid gland and sexual gland; or hyperfunction of the pancreatic adrenal cortex. These patients need diagnosis and treatment from medical professionals to first tackle the primary diseases. This is not a simple problem of weight loss.

According to traditional Chinese medicine, even gentle physical activity would make obese people short of breath and accelerate their heartbeat. Therefore, they are unwilling to move much. Thus a vicious cycle occurs. They become fatter and fatter, and prone to various chronic diseases. For example, they tend to further develop from hyperlipidemia and vascular sclerosis to hypertension, diabetes, cardio-cerebral-vascular system diseases, fatty liver and psychological disorders. Longevity may also be affected. Achieving weight loss has a true medical rationale, rather than just the motivation of becoming more physically attractive.

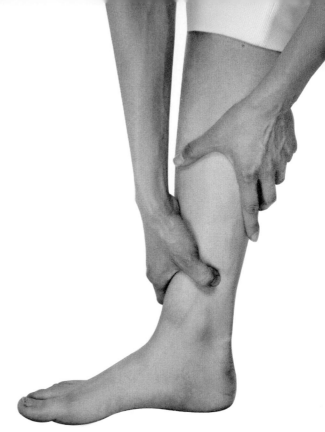

Pinch and rub the Sanyinjiao point.

Meridian and Collateral Exercises

Please spend about twenty minutes every day practicing all the sixteen steps of the exercises for tapping meridians and collaterals. You can also choose the following six steps from among the sixteen, practicing them coherently or separately. Practice them once to twice a day, gradually increasing repetitions.

1. Step 3 hand-throwing and tiptoeing: 200 to 500 times
2. Waist rotation of Step 6: 50 to 100 times
3. Step 13 pushing a "wall": four 8-beats
4. Tapping the Qihai point and Mingmen point of Step 14: applying more force with your hand for four 8-beats
5. Tapping on and along the spine of Step 14: applying more force with your hand and moving up and down the spine for four sequences of four 8-beats
6. Step 15 swaying and shaking: 1 to 3 minutes

Self-Massaging

1. Acupoint pinching and rubbing of the Zusanli point, Sanyinjiao point, Yongquan point: Apply force anti-clockwise to pinch and rub. 3 to 5 minutes, once to twice a day.

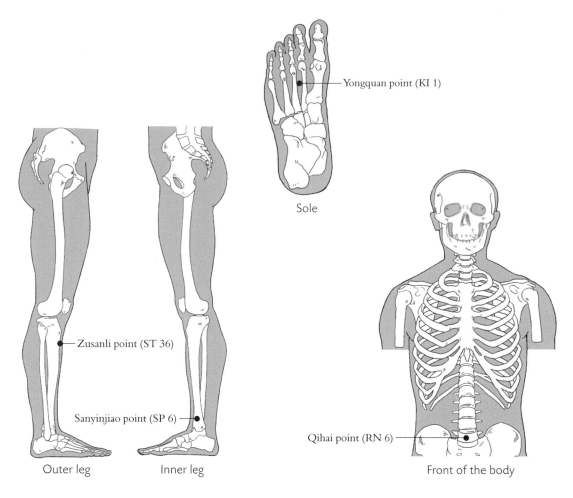

Yongquan point (KI 1)

Sole

Zusanli point (ST 36)

Sanyinjiao point (SP 6)

Outer leg   Inner leg

Qihai point (RN 6)

Front of the body

2. Abdomen pushing and pressing: Overlap your palms and place them on your abdomen. Apply force clockwise around your Qihai point, pushing and pressing your abdomen. 300 to 500 circles, once to twice a day.

Additional Tips

1. Aerobic exercise: This should be approached scientifically, choosing exercises based on consumption of body fat, i.e. low-intensity and long-term exercises. Exercise once a day or every other day.

2. Control heart rate: During exercises, keep the heart rate at less than 120 times per minute, and gradually extend the period of exercise to over 45 minutes. If the duration is too short, the glycogen reserved in the muscles can provide enough energy, and fat will not be burned; instead the exercise may just increase the appetite.

3. Choosing suitable activities: It is easiest to stick with an exercise program if you choose activities (e.g., fast walk, jogging, swimming, dancing, etc.) that suit your interests and strengths.

4. Gradual approach: Obese people may have relatively weak heart and lung functions and a poorer physique. Therefore they should do exercises according to their ability and increase step by step, gradually prolonging the duration and increasing the frequency. This is the only way to lose weight safely and effectively.

2 Hyperlipidemia

Hyperlipidemia refers to the increase of fats in the blood plasma; it usually refers to one or more of the following: the increase of the total cholesterol, triglycerides and/or low-density lipoprotein, or the decline of high-density lipoprotein. Hyperlipidemia may be primary, thus causing other diseases. It can also be the symptom of another disease such as hypertension, diabetes, coronary heart disease or endocrine system disease. These influence each other and form a vicious cycle. You can mitigate the harm of hyperlipidemia to your health through the following healthcare methods.

Meridian and Collateral Exercises

Please spend about 20 minutes every day practicing all sixteen steps of the meridian and collateral exercises in Chapter Two. You can also choose the following from among these sixteen steps to practice together or separately, moderately increasing the times of repetition. You should develop a habit of practicing them at least once to twice every day.

1. Step 3 hand-throwing and tiptoeing: 100 to 200 times
2. Push and rub your chest and abdomen of Step 9: four 8-beats
3. Tapping the Qihai point and Mingmen point of Step 14: applying more force with your hand, four 8-beats
4. Tapping on and along the spine of Step 14: applying more force with your hand; moving up and down, and side to side for four times of four 8-beats
5. Step 13 pushing a "wall": four 8-beats

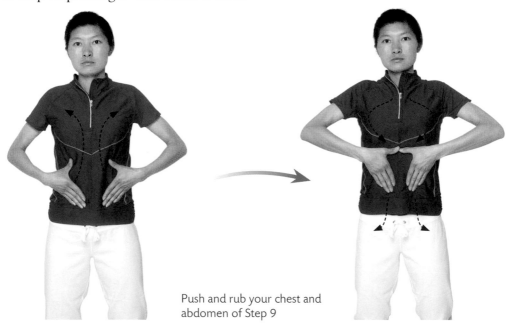

Push and rub your chest and abdomen of Step 9

Self-Massaging

1. Acupoint pinching and rubbing of the Zusanli point, Sanyinjiao point and Yongquan point: Apply force to pinch and rub in a counterclockwise direction for three to five minutes, once to twice a day.

2. Abdomen pushing and pressing: Overlap your palms and place them on your abdomen. Around your Qihai point, apply force clockwise and counterclockwise to push and press your abdomen for 100 to 200 circles, once to twice a day.

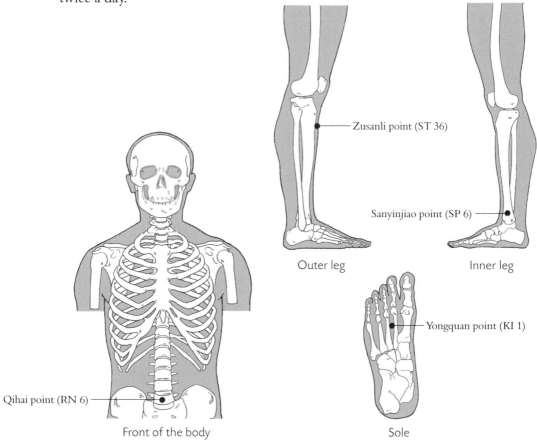

Zusanli point (ST 36)

Sanyinjiao point (SP 6)

Outer leg   Inner leg

Yongquan point (KI 1)

Qihai point (RN 6)

Front of the body   Sole

Additional Tips

1. Abide by the principle of a balanced diet: eat fewer desserts; do not show particular preference for certain foods; and do not eat snacks.

2. Vinegar therapy: This method has been circulated in China as a folk remedy for a long time, however it is unsuitable for sufferers of such diseases as hyperacidity and gastric ulcer. Mix 50 ml of food-quality vinegar with 500–1000 ml water. Drink a small amount often. Do not directly drink undiluted vinegar, which can harm the gastric mucosa. You can also achieve the same effect by adding some vinegar to your everyday meals, consuming about one spoonful in your food every day. Moreover drinking a little vinegar water after exercise can help relieve muscular ache and fatigue, and promote the restoration of your physical strength.

3 Insomnia

Insomnia can be a reaction caused by a neurological disorder or it can be the symptom of a disease. Insomniacs have problems in getting enough sleep or in falling asleep, and tend to be restless during sleep. Long-term insomnia can bring about a series of problems, including fatigue, dizziness, poor appetite, abnormal mood, inattention, forgetfulness and decline of mental capacity, and other functional or even pathological changes. In addition, insomnia will further affect your health and reduce your resistance to disease. There are many traditional Chinese therapies against insomnia such as herbal remedies, however the focus here is on tapping and self-massaging.

Meridian and Collateral Exercises

Please spend about twenty minutes every day practicing all the sixteen steps of the meridian and collateral exercises in Chapter Two. You can also choose the following to practice coherently or separately, and moderately increase repetitions. Complete these steps while lying down on a bed.

1. Ear-lifting of Step 10: four 8-beats on the left and the right side respectively
2. Step 8 combing and scraping: four 8-beats
3. Push and rub your face of Step 9: four 8-beats

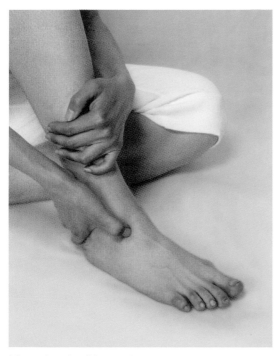

Massaging the Qiuxu point

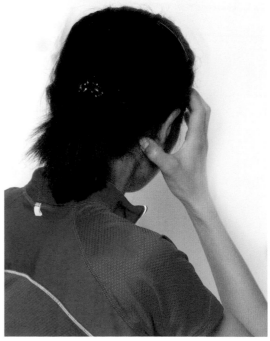

Massaging the Yiming point

Self-Massaging

Choose any of the following acupoints, and pinch and rub each point for 1 to 2 minutes, once a day before bed.

1. Acupoints in the feet: Yongquan point, Lidui point, Taixi point, Qiuxu point, Xingjian point

2. Acupoints in the four limbs and head: Sanyinjiao point, Shenmen point, Baihui point, Yiming point

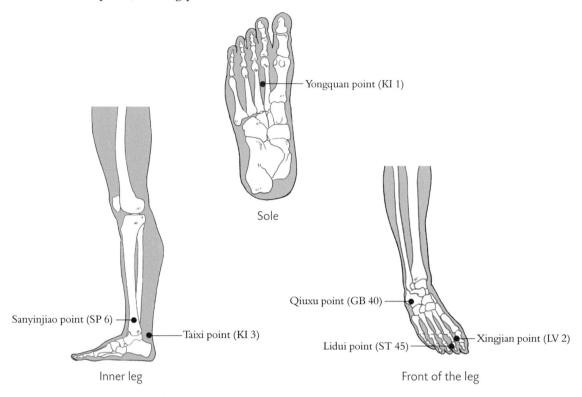

Yongquan point (KI 1)

Sole

Sanyinjiao point (SP 6)

Taixi point (KI 3)

Inner leg

Qiuxu point (GB 40)

Lidui point (ST 45)

Xingjian point (LV 2)

Front of the leg

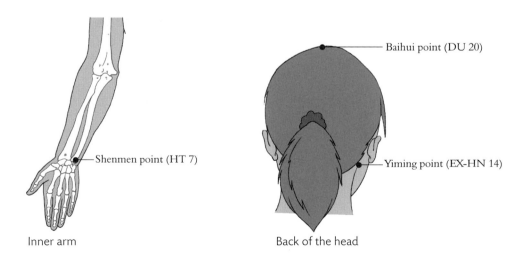

Shenmen point (HT 7)

Inner arm

Baihui point (DU 20)

Yiming point (EX-HN 14)

Back of the head

Additional Exercise: Breath-Regulation Before Bed

This method is an important part of preventing and treating insomnia. Breath-regulation therapy before sleep refers to balancing yin and yang in your body by regulating qi activity during breathing. It is an important part of the healthcare science of traditional Chinese medicine. TCM holds that health can be maintained and diseases prevented only by keeping brisk vitality within body. This "vitality" includes the coordination of nerve centers and various systems of the body, the stability of resistance, keeping a positive outlook and tranquil mind, and the smooth operation of metabolism and physiological functions. Through this can life be prolonged.

Studies of the brain have shown that practicing breath-regulation can strengthen the inhibitory state of the cerebral cortex, and weaken the unusually excited state. This therapy can not only serve as an adjuvant therapy for insomnia caused by various factors, but it can also regulate the physical and mental state of people who do not suffer from insomnia, to improve their sleep.

The main points of this therapy include "passing three steps" and "choosing three postures."

1. "Passing three barriers": You must first grasp three main points: i.e. you need to adjust your posture, regulate your breathing, and regulate your mind.

Step 1: Adjust Your Posture
Whichever posture you choose, you should first relax your whole body. When you feel comfortable all over your body, without any conflicts within, you have relaxed yourself thoroughly.

Step 2: Regulate Your Breath
Change from your customary thoracic respiration to abdominal breathing. Imagine the air inhaled as it goes into your nasal cavity, passes

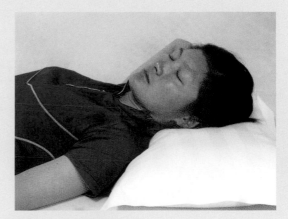

Adjust your posture.

through your chest, and reaches your lower abdomen. At this time your abdomen will rise.

Towards the end of your inhalation, gently lift your anus, i.e. contract your anal sphincter. Then imagine retracting the lower abdomen to press the air back to your chest. Then the air can be gently exhaled through your mouth. You should loosen from the groin at the same time.

When commencing this technique, it is recommended that you place your palm at the center of your lower abdomen, so that you can feel, and not only image, its movement. This will allow you to regulate the smoothness and rhythm of the abdominal respiration more naturally and thoroughly. Beginners should first start from natural rhythmic breathing and gradually turn it into gentle and slow deep breathing.

By reinforcing the interaction of the muscles of the diaphragm, abdomen and perineum, this kind of abdominal respiration can gently, slowly and rhythmically change the inner pressure of abdomen. This will produce a continuous and gentle massage over all organs in the abdomen, including the liver, gallbladder, pancreas, spleen, kidney, urinary tract and gastrointestinal tract, and even the adrenal gland, male prostate, testis, female ovary, uterus and other endocrine and reproductive organs.

By improving the blood circulation of the abdomen, abdominal respiration can improve the functions of all the above mentioned body parts. In addition due to the increase of the volume of blood flowing back to the heart, abdominal respiration can improve blood circulation in the entire body. Furthermore since the rising and falling amplitude of the diaphragm is greater during abdominal respiration than during thoracic respiration, abdominal respiration can also increase lung capacity and the supply of blood and oxygen, and considerably improve metabolism.

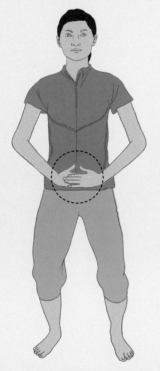

It is generally thought that there are upper, central and lower elixir fields in the human body. The upper elixir refers to the brain; the central elixir refers to the heart; and the lower elixir refers to the center of lower abdomen. The general term "elixir field" refers to the lower elixir field. TCM regards essence, qi and spirit as the body's three treasures. They are concealed in the lower, central and upper elixir field respectively.

Step 3: Regulate Your Mind

The mind is intangible and abstract. Therefore this is the most difficult step. However it embodies the highest realm of the breath-regulation therapy, so you should practice this step repeatedly and devotedly.

According to TCM, the mind controls all mental activities, including cogitation, spirit and mood. The key to regulating the mind is to applying control to concentrate your attention as soon as possible on your elixir field (*dantian*). You should relax quietly and then naturally enter a state of "nihility." In other words, you should enter a state in which you think about nothing. In this way, you can complete the step of regulating your mind.

To help accomplish this, use the following visualization technique. Concentrate your attention on the undulating feeling under your palm when you breathe abdominally. You can imagine that it is a wave rising up and down. You will feel as if you are lying on a small boat, drifting with the wave, surrounded by blue sky and white clouds, green trees, soaring birds and gentle breezes. In this way you will gradually drift from a state of quietness to a state of nihility, and slowly go into your dream.

During practice, do not strive for success; otherwise you will become restless and it will be difficult for you to still yourself. You need to practice this step slowly and understand it earnestly.

Traditional Chinese medicine lays particular emphasis on spiritual maintenance. Here "spirit" broadly encompasses the "seven emotions," including various thinking and mental activities. TCM specifically regards the seven emotions as being closely related to the physiological and pathological changes of the five internal organs. It warns people not to indulge their emotions too much otherwise these five internal organs may be damaged. Some traditional beliefs include: "rage impairs liver; delight impairs heart; anxiety impairs spleen; sorrow impairs lung; fright impairs kidney."

Only by regulating your spirit into a peaceful state can you maintain the dynamic balance of yin and yang in your body, clear your qi and blood, pacify your internal organs, and keep energy and health, maintaining distance from illness. A vital part of breath-regulation therapy, "regulating your mind" is the best method for nourishing and maintaining your spirit, which has tremendous health benefits.

2. "Choosing three postures": During the exercises of this therapy, three basic postures are usually adopted: standing, sitting and reclining. The posture of reclining will be thoroughly explained in the following, and further includes three postures: lying on the back, lying on the side, and lying on the back with legs crossed. You are free to choose one of these postures or practice the three postures in turn according to your own preference.

Posture 1: Lying on the Back

Lie horizontally on the bed. A thin pillow should be used, preferably stuffed with buckwheat husk, packed loosely, so that you can change its thickness and shape as you wish.

Cross your legs or naturally separate them (the latter is preferable). Relax your whole body, close your eyes, support your upper palate gently with the tip of your tongue, smile and cross both your palms, putting them at the center of your lower abdomen.

In order to mitigate the pressure of your arms on your abdomen during abdominal respiration, you can fix your elbows to provide support at the end of deep inhalation. In this way you will feel much more comfortable.

Posture 2: Lying on the Back Cross-Legged

This is a new posture I invented during practice. It can be applied the most often, especially during short-term breaks.

Buddhist monks often sit cross-legged during meditation. This action can promote flexibility. In particular, due to long-term stretching, the muscles and ligaments on the inner side of the thigh and in the groin and hip can become more supple, thus considerably enhancing flexibility during activities and reducing athletic injury.

Moreover in the process of cross-legged sitting, the distance between the legs and heart is shortened, improving blood circulation in the limbs and helping to cure pain in the joints of the lower limbs. In the process of lying down, the muscles stretched during cross-legged sitting can continue to be pulled, and the quadriceps femoris muscle in the front of thigh also is stretched. In addition this position can reduce the stress on the waist and back that can occur from long-term cross-legged sitting.

Please note that it is somewhat difficult to lie on the back cross-legged. Beginners can persist for only a few minutes but will be able to gradually extend the time of their practice. After a feeling of numbness occurs, it is best to adopt the position of lying on the back instead. Don't rush into over-practicing this difficult posture; with time you should be able to remain in the position for 30 to 40 minutes without undue stress. Please note that while changing positions it is best to first straighten one foot slowly, and then the other. Changing too quickly can strain your hip joint.

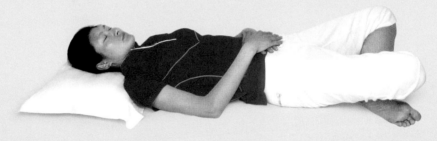

Lie on the back cross-legged.

Posture 3: Lying on the Side

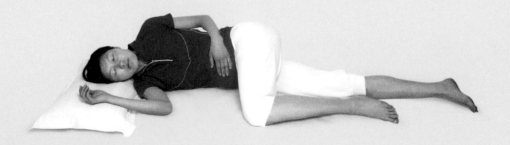

Lie on your right side. Adjust the pillow with your hand so it is as thick as the width of your right shoulder, which will mitigate the sense of pressure of your head and face. Straighten your right leg and cross your left leg over it, bending it so that it is also on the bed. Bend your left arm and place your left palm at the center of your lower abdomen. Bend your right arm and stretch it outward naturally, placing the back of your right palm on the pillow.

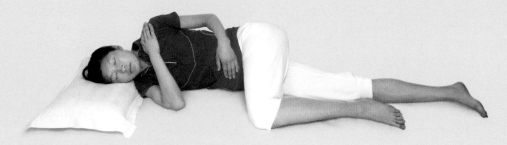

Or bend your right arm toward your chest, and support your left shoulder with your right palm.

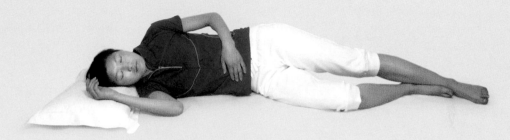

You can also bend your right leg, and then straighten your left leg and place it on your right ankle. Bend your left arm and place your left palm at the center of your lower abdomen.

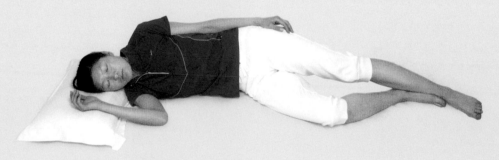

Or straighten your left arm and place it on your left leg.

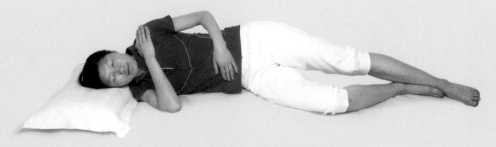

You can keep your right arm in the above-mentioned posture. Bend it and stretch it outward naturally, placing the back of your palm on the pillow. Or bend your right arm toward your chest, then support your left shoulder with your right palm.

4 General Malaise

General malaise is defined in TCM as a reaction to the decline of your physical ability and the functions of your organs. It can also be the premonitory symptom of a disease. Only common fatigue is discussed here, including fatigue caused by excessive mental and physical activities.

Fatigue is not a disease. It refers to constraint of physical ability, decline of organ functions, frequent feeling of tiredness, lack of strength and possibly other accompanying discomforts. Moreover different people may have quite different manifestations. However sufferers will neither have any physical problem upon physical examination nor any clinical objective indication.

Please note that many diseases can be accompanied by the symptom of general malaise as they develop and therefore would indeed be accompanied by some clinical indications related to the primary disease. However this does not fall within the scope of this book.

Meridian and Collateral Exercises

Please spend about 20 minutes every day practicing all the sixteen steps of the meridian and collateral exercises in Chapter Two. You can also choose the following steps from the sixteen to practice coherently or separately, once or twice a day. Over time you can moderately increase the repetitions.

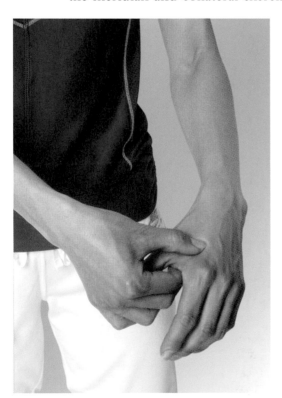

Pinch and rub your Hegu point.

1. Ear-lifting of Step 10: on the left and right side respectively, four 8-beats

2. Tapping the Qihai point and Mingmen point of Step 14: four 8-beats

3. Tapping on and along the spine of Step 14: up and down and back and forth for four times of four 8-beats

4. Push and rub your chest and abdomen of Step 9: four 8-beats

5. Step 16 closing eyes meditatively: 3 to 5 minutes

Self-Massaging

Gently pinch and rub your Hegu point, Neiguan point, Zusanli point and Sanyinjiao point clockwise; 1 to 2 minutes for each point, once to twice a day.

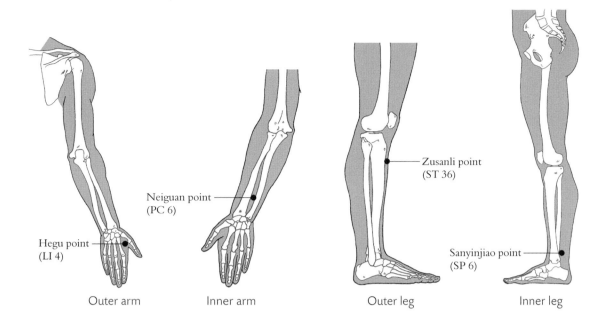

Outer arm   Inner arm   Outer leg   Inner leg

Hegu point (LI 4)

Neiguan point (PC 6)

Zusanli point (ST 36)

Sanyinjiao point (SP 6)

Additional Tips

You should commence with easy exercises, medium-speed walking, dancing or light calistentics. In addition you need to abide by a schedule, refrain from smoking, limit drinking, balance your diet and remain optimistic.

5 | Cold Hands and Feet

Usually people who have cold hands also have cold feet, and they are sensitive to the change of air temperature. Even in the morning and evening of hot days they may feel cold in their hands and feet, and the temperature of their hands and feet is always lower than that of ordinary people. This symptom is more prevalent among females.

In fact this is a common manifestation of weak micro-circulation, and it is directly related to the decline of pumping force of the cardiac muscle and the decrease of cardiac output. When the cardiac output declines, the blood flowing toward the ends of the four limbs decreases, micro-circulation becomes insufficient, and metabolism slows down. Therefore the temperature in some parts of body declines. If this goes on for a very long time, it inevitably has a negative effect on the functions of various body systems.

According to TCM, this is a manifestation of the deficiency of qi, especially yang qi, and is regarded as a sign of disease. People with deficient qi will surely not have smooth blood vessels, and as time goes by, blood stasis and illness occur.

Of course cold hands and feet can also be related to diseases or states of nutrition, e.g. the inflammation of some blood vessels, spasms, obstructions, necrosis and other pathological changes, peripheral neuritis, etc. Therefore you should pay attention to the phenomena of your own cold hands and feet, and take steps to rectify it over time.

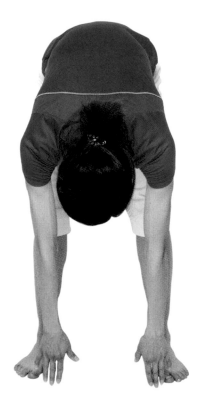

Bend your waist and touch the ground of Step 11

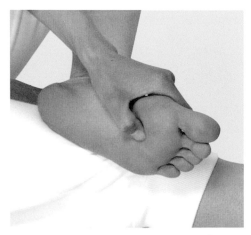

Pinch and rub your Yongquan point clockwise.

Meridian and Collateral Exercises

You should spend about 20 minutes every day practicing all sixteen steps of the meridian and collateral exercises in Chapter Two. You can also choose the following steps to practice coherently or separately, once to twice a day, moderately increasing repetitions over time.

1. Step 3 hand-throwing and tiptoeing: 100 to 200 times; this will produce good effects instantly.

2. Tapping the Qihai point and Mingmen point of Step 14: four 8-beats

3. Tapping the buttocks and the outer thigh and calf of Step 14: four 8-beats

4. Tapping the inside of the thigh and calf of Step 14: four 8-beats

5. Tapping on and along the spine of Step 14: up and down and back and forth, 50 times

6. Step 12 letting go and taking in breath: four 8-beats

7. Step 13 pushing a "wall": four 8-beats

8. Bend your waist and touch the ground of Step 11: four 8-beats

9. Step 15 swaying and shaking: 2 to 3 minutes

Self-Massaging

Apply force clockwise to pinch and rub your Yongquan point, Taichong point, Zusanli point and Hegu point; 1 to 2 minutes for each point, once to twice a day.

Additional Tips

1. Increase aerobic exercise: It is best to use a moderate walking pace, developing a good habit of walking 130 to 150 steps within 60 to 70 seconds while covering a distance of about 100 meters. You should walk at least 30 minutes at a stretch, 3 to 4 times a week.

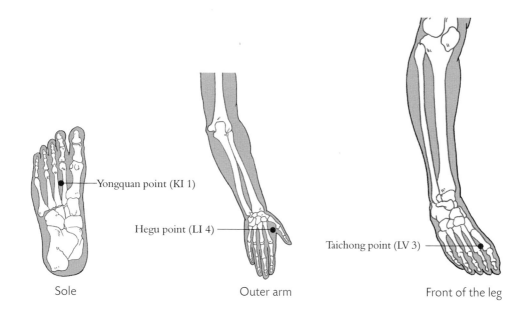

Yongquan point (KI 1)

Hegu point (LI 4)

Taichong point (LV 3)

Sole   Outer arm   Front of the leg

The main points to keep in mind about this kind of "healthcare walk" are to raise your head, swing your arms high, walk at a moderate pace, breathe deeply, and clench your fists to involve your hands. This will enhance the walking exercise by involving both the upper and lower limbs. It can effectively increase the volume of pulmonary ventilation and improve heart and lung functions and micro-circulation.

In addition to walking, you can choose other outdoor aerobic exercises such as jogging, hiking, boating, body-building exercises or tai chi (*taijiquan*).

2. Rub your hands together rapidly: Cross your ten fingers, suspend both arms in the air, and rub your hands together rapidly and continuously. Although this may seem simple, the majority of people cannot persist for one minute. Only by rubbing your hands together continually for one minute, at a frequency of more than 180 times, can you achieve a good effect.

Almost all meridians and collaterals distributed on the hands meet one another on both sides of the fingertips. Therefore rubbing your hands in this way can not only clear your meridians and collaterals but also strengthen the force of your arm muscles and obviously improve the micro-circulation of your hands. Older people with chronic diseases and weak physique should rub their hands at a lower speed in case of any discomfort.

3. Raise the tip of your toes: When sitting for a long time, every 20 minutes you can strongly and repeatedly raise the tip of your toes 20 to 30 times, which will help improve the micro-circulation of your feet.

4. Frequently eat ginger slices and jujubes soaked in vinegar: You can eat them as snacks during three daily regular meals. These foods help warm your meridians and tonify your qi. Therefore they can improve your micro-circulation.

5. Keep warm, in particular your four limbs: Bathe your feet or your whole body in hot water for 10 to 15 minutes before sleep.

6 | Visual Fatigue

Visual fatigue is a common eye problem, and may include the inability to focus on nearby objects for a long time; sore eyes; blurred vision; dry eyes; lachrymation (tearing up of the eyes); or even headache, nausea, dizziness, etc. There are many causes of visual fatigue, however only following causes are discussed here: long-term computer use; long-term sedentary work; working with something at a close distance; and excessive regulation and tension of the eyes.

You should regulate the intensity of your work and study, use your eyes for only a moderate length of time without a break, and work and study under reasonable illumination. If you are near-sighted be sure to choose suitable glasses and often gaze at objects in the distance.

Meridian and Collateral Exercises

The following steps have been chosen from among the set of sixteen meridian and collateral exercises. Please practice them once to twice a day.

1. Eye rotation of Step 6: rotating to the left and the right for two 8-beats respectively

2. Step 2 holding a "ball" in a horse-riding stance: two 8-beats

3. Step 7 pinching and rubbing: four times of four 8-beats

4. Push and rub your face of Step 9: four 8-beats

Self-Massaging

Please pinch and rub your Taiyang point, Yintang point, Cuanzhu point, Sizhukong point, Jingming point, Sibai point and Fengchi point; 1 to 2 minutes for each point, once to twice a day.

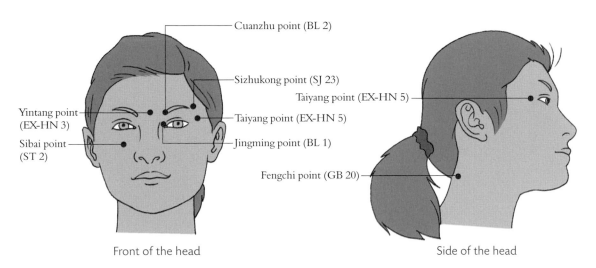

Cuanzhu point (BL 2)

Sizhukong point (SJ 23)

Taiyang point (EX-HN 5)

Yintang point (EX-HN 3)

Taiyang point (EX-HN 5)

Sibai point (ST 2)

Jingming point (BL 1)

Fengchi point (GB 20)

Front of the head   Side of the head

7 | Loss of Appetite

Loss of appetite has the following manifestations: no desire to eat; inability to eat at mealtime; and decrease of food intake. Common causes include diseases and the administration of certain drugs as well fatigue, including excessive mental or physical activities. In addition, bad living habits, such as over-eating, dietary bias, irregular dining, eating too much raw or cold food, excessive intake of beverages and the misuse of healthcare products are also causes of loss of appetite.

Meridian and Collateral Exercises

Please spend about 20 minutes every day practicing all the sixteen steps of the meridian and collateral exercises in Chapter Two. The following steps, practiced coherently or separately, are also beneficial. Practice them once to twice a day, moderately increase repetition over time.

1. Step 5 teeth-clicking and swallowing: clicking teeth 100 times

2. Tapping the Qihai point and Mingmen point of Step 14: four 8-beats

3. Tapping on and along the spine of Step 14: up and down and back and forth, four times of four 8-beats

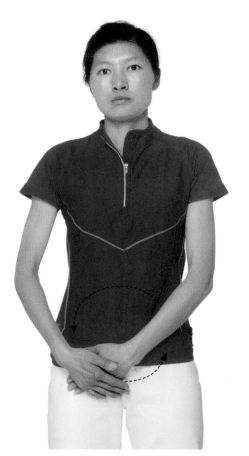

Push and rub the abdomen.

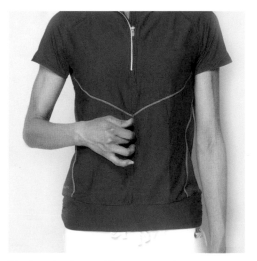

Pinch and rub your Zhongwan point.

Self-Massaging

1. Pinching and rubbing your Zusanli point, Zhongwan point, Qihai point and Neiguan point: 1 to 2 minutes for each point, once to twice a day.

2. Push and rub your abdomen: 100 to 200 circles clockwise and counterclockwise respectively, once to twice a day.

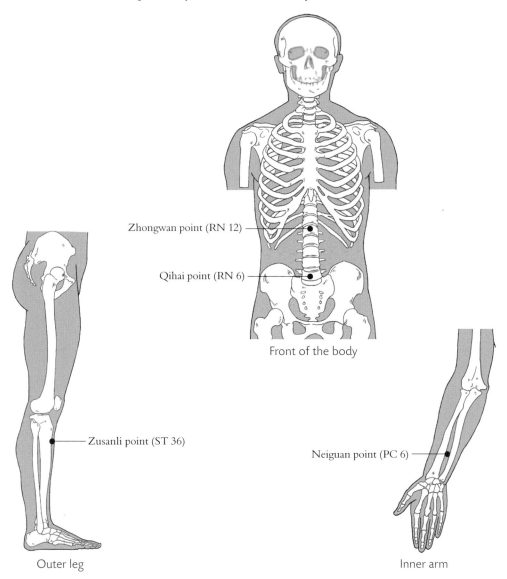

Zhongwan point (RN 12)

Qihai point (RN 6)

Front of the body

Zusanli point (ST 36)

Neiguan point (PC 6)

Outer leg

Inner arm

Additional Tips

Please actively eliminate causes of loss of appetite, and improve cuisine, change your tastes and moderately choose a little spicy food and other food with pungent tastes. Reinforce aerobic exercises, e.g. walking, jogging, hiking, boating, body-building exercises, tai chi, etc.

8 Mental Stress

Mental stress is mostly caused by emergency situations or due to long-term pressures from life, work, study, diseases, etc. Its manifestations include being overwhelmed or having an unstable mood, irritableness, anxiety, difficulty going to sleep or disturbed sleep, lassitude, forgetfulness, distraction and other mental abnormities. These can further produce nervous disorders such as digestive dysfunction, headache, dizziness, hidrosis (excessive sweating), numb limbs, and ache and pain of the whole body. However no physical root cause will be found out in most cases.

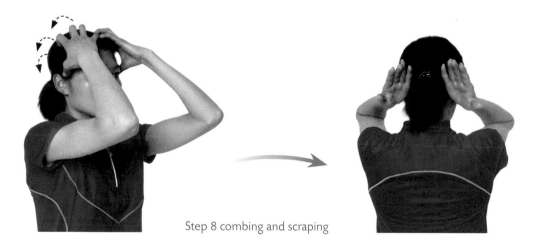

Step 8 combing and scraping

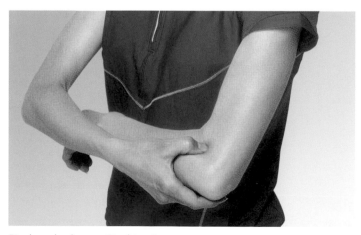

Pinch and rub your Quchi point.

10 | Constipation

Constipation refers to dry or problematic defecation, often caused by improper living habits such as unsuitable diet. This may include too little fiber or vegetables and fruits, too much meat, insufficient water intake, and preference for spicy and hot foods. Other causes include lack of activity, irregular timing of defecation, and hasty or distracted defecation. In addition to focusing on eliminating these problems, you can use self-healthcare method to relieve constipation.

Meridian and Collateral Exercises

Please spend about 20 minutes every day practicing all the sixteen steps of meridian and collateral exercises, and add, separately or coherently, the following steps to practice once to twice a day. Moderately increase the times of repetition.

1. Teeth-clicking of Step 5: 100 times
2. Hip rotation of Step 6: left and right, four 8-beats respectively
3. Push and rub your chest and abdomen of Step 9: 100 to 200 circles clockwise around your navel
4. Step 13 pushing a "wall": four 8-beats
5. Tapping the Qihai point and Mingmen point of Step 14: applying more force than usual for four 8-beats
6. Tapping on and along the spine of Step 14: using more force than usual to tap up and down and back and forth, four times of four 8-beats

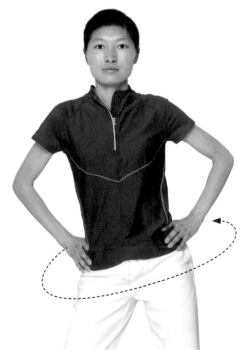

Hip rotation of Step 6

Self-Massaging

Pinch and rub your Shenque point, Qihai point, Tianshu point, Guanyuan point and Zusanli point: counterclockwise for 2 to 3 minutes, once to twice a day. The massaged points are the same as those selected for diarrhea. However the points are gently pressed and rubbed clockwise for diarrhea while they are forcefully pressed and rubbed counterclockwise for constipation.

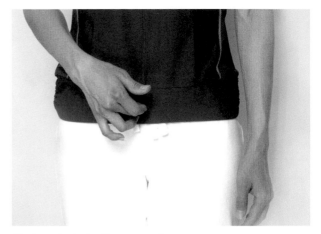

Pinch and rub the Shenque point.

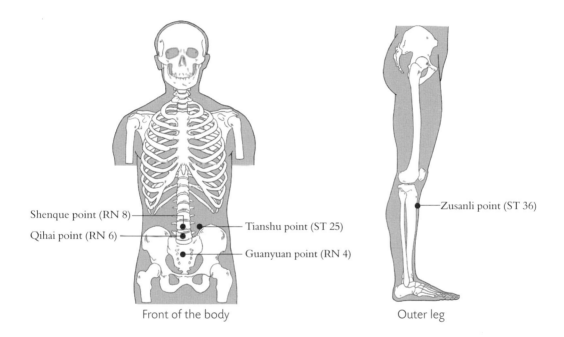

Shenque point (RN 8)
Qihai point (RN 6)
Tianshu point (ST 25)
Guanyuan point (RN 4)

Front of the body

Zusanli point (ST 36)

Outer leg

Additional Tips

1. Dietary suggestion: Eat more fruits and vegetables while taking in less spicy and hot food. Drink more water and do more physical exercises.

2. Changing bathroom habits: Do not read while defecating so as not to distract your attention and inhibit your defecation reflex. Learn to use abdominal respiration while defecating. Do not try to produce force with your belly repeatedly. This may cause the inner pressure of your chest and abdomen to increase suddenly, thus bringing potential risks to patients with cardiovascular or hemorrhagic diseases, or hemorrhoids, slowly weakening the active contracting ability of your intestinal tract during defecation and causing or aggravating constipation.

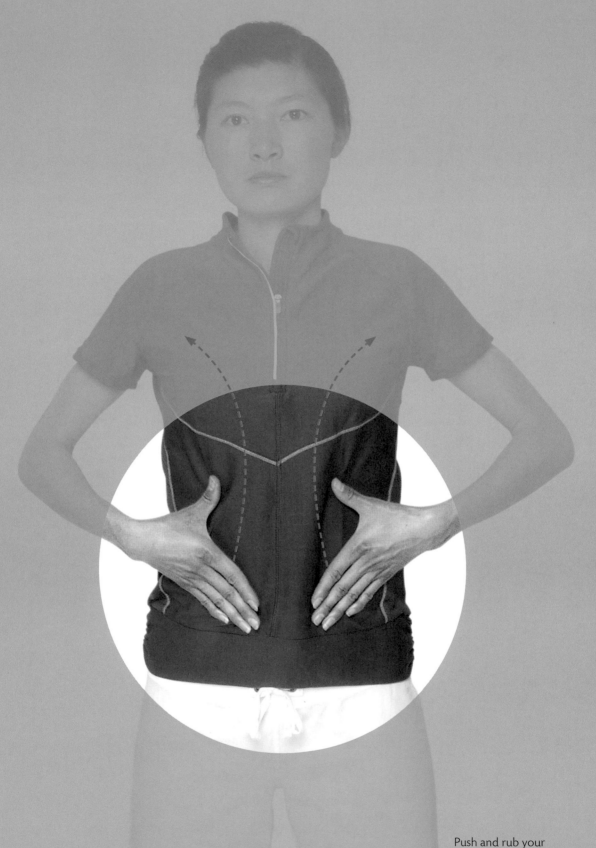

Push and rub your
chest and abdomen
of Step 9 on page 43

CHAPTER FIVE
Meridian and Collateral Methods for Chronic Diseases

This chapter looks at 19 common diseases, focusing on the non-clinical but very effective treatments developed from the experience I have accumulated in practicing clinical and sports medicine over the past forty years. Of course, these traditional or folk remedies are not a replacement for medical consultation and treatment. However, as long as you understand your condition and symptoms, the diligent application of these methods will result in surprising and real therapeutic effects.

1 Hypertension

The increase of blood pressure is common. If the blood pressure of an adult is higher than or equal to 140/90 mm Hg during three different measurements on the same day, this can be diagnosed as hypertension.

Hypertension includes primary and secondary hypertension, with the former being more common. It refers to the continuous increase of the arterial blood pressure caused by sclerosis and abnormal nervous regulation of the vasomotor center. The latter can be caused by diabetes; kidney, endocrine or other diseases; or as the side effect of drugs. During treatment, the underlying diseases must be treated first.

Drugs for curing hypertension must be taken systematically, maintaining a constant dosage. Moreover, one must not stop taking the drugs suddenly. It must be understood that the methods introduced here are only suitable for mild and moderate hypertension patients on the basis of systematic treatment.

Meridian and Collateral Healthcare Exercises

Please spend about 20 minutes every day practicing all the sixteen steps of the meridian and collateral exercises in Chapter Two. To treat hypertension you may choose the following steps from among these sixteen steps. Practice them coherently or separately, once to twice a day, gradually increasing repetitions.

1. Step 3 throwing and tiptoeing: 50 to 100 times; the action can be slower
2. Step 8 combing and scraping: four 8-beats
3. Step 7 pinching and rubbing: four 8-beats, repeated four times
4. Tapping on and along the spine of Step 14: four repetitions of four 8-beats; you can tap more gently
5. Step 15 swaying and shaking: 2 to 3 minutes
6. Step 16 closing eyes meditatively: 2 to 3 minutes

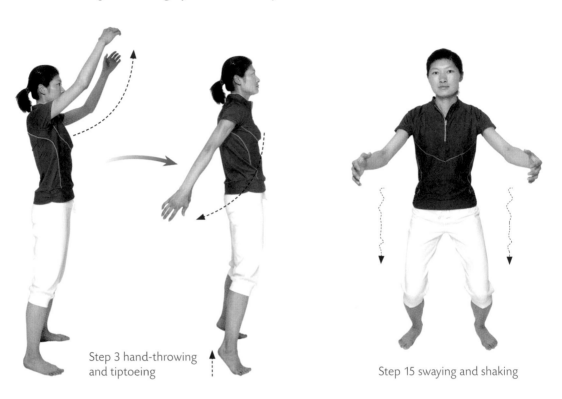

Step 3 hand-throwing and tiptoeing

Step 15 swaying and shaking

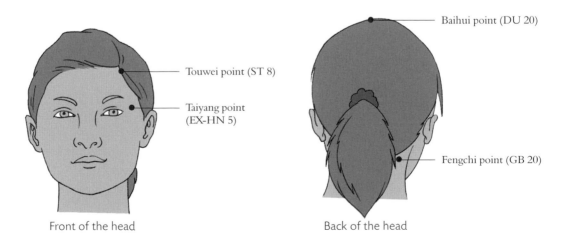

Touwei point (ST 8)

Taiyang point (EX-HN 5)

Baihui point (DU 20)

Fengchi point (GB 20)

Front of the head

Back of the head

Self-Massaging

Pinch and rub your Touwei point, Taiyang point, Baihui point, Fengchi point, Neiguan point and Sanyinjiao point. 1 to 2 minutes for each point, once to twice a day.

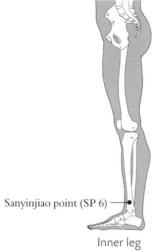

Sanyinjiao point (SP 6)

Inner leg

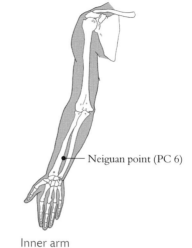

Neiguan point (PC 6)

Inner arm

Additional Tips

1. Choose low-intensity aerobic exercises and relaxation techniques of various types. These may include walking, jogging, dancing, aerobics, yoga, tai chi, table tennis, strength training with light weights, and different kinds of relaxation training. You can alternate between two or three of these methods according to your personal preferences.

2. Reduce or avoid exercises that constrain breathing, and exercises during which the head is lower than the waist.

3. Take the exercises step by step, observing any changes of blood pressure, and making any necessary adjustments. If you do not feel tired and your blood pressure remains stable, and you feel full of energy and spirit the next morning, this is a sign that you can continue to do these exercises.

4. Contraindications: Discontinue the exercises when your blood pressure is not effectively controlled or is unstable. You must stop immediately if any serious complications that impair your heart, brain, kidney or other target organs occur, or if symptoms indicating the aggravation of your disease occur, e.g. dizziness, headache, cardiac arrhythmia, choking sensation in the chest, and angina. In these cases you need to consult a doctor, and may then continue with light indoor or in-bed exercises.

5. Other prevention and treatment techniques: Non-medical techniques—such as listening to light music; refraining from smoking and drinking; lowering intake of salt, sugar and fat; taking in a high content of vitamins and a moderate content of protein—are also important. It is also recommended to drink broadleaf holly leaf tea, oolong tea or Tieguanyin tea. Pay attention to your mental health and take steps to relieve your tension. It is also important to effectively reduce and control your body fat and weight (see the "obesity" section in Chapter Four).

2 Diabetes

Diabetes is a common disease, and its prevalence rate has been growing worldwide. Diabetes refers to a metabolic disorder characterized by chronic hyperglycemia. Long-term diabetes can bring about multi-system damage, e.g. chronic progressive deterioration of the eyes, kidneys, nerves, heart, blood vessels and other tissues, and can bring about functional defect and failure.

Currently it is thought that diabetes is the syndrome of compound etiological factors, and is related to such factors as heredity, autoimmunity and environment. Treatment includes comprehensive measures in the following five aspects: diet, drugs, exercise, health education and self-monitoring. The functions of exercise intervention include: reducing blood sugar, lipids and pressure; increasing energy consumption; reducing weight; retarding insulin resistance; regulating and controlling insulin secretion; and delaying the genesis and development of complications. In particular regarding diabetes, exercise intervention plays an important role in reducing the risks of atherosclerotic cardiovascular diseases.

The following methods of self-treatment introduced here can be used by patients with mild and moderate diabetes as part of systematic treatment.

Meridian and Collateral Exercises

Please spend about 20 minutes every day practicing all sixteen steps of meridian and collateral exercises in Chapter Two. You can also choose the

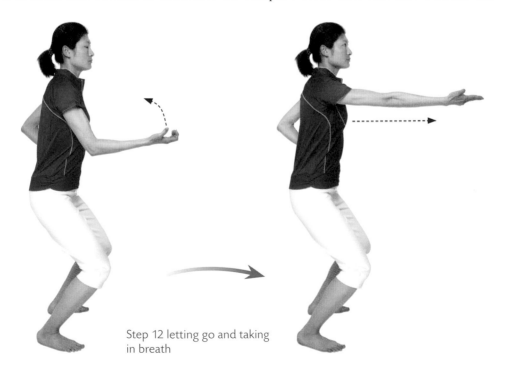

Step 12 letting go and taking in breath

following steps to practice together or separately, once to twice a day. Moderately increase the times of repetition.

1. Step 3 hand-throwing and tiptoeing: 50 to 100 times
2. Step 12 letting go and taking in breath: four 8-beats
3. Step 13 pushing a "wall": four 8-beats; if you cannot squat fully, please semi-squat.
4. Tapping the inside of the thigh and calf of Step 14: four 8-beats
5. Tapping on and along the spine of Step 14: up and down, and side to side for four times of four 8-beats
6. Step 15 swaying and shaking: 3 to 5 minutes

Self-Massaging

Gently pinch and rub your Zusanli, Sanyinjiao, Shenshu, Pishu and Geshu points: 1 to 2 minutes for each point, twice to three times a day.

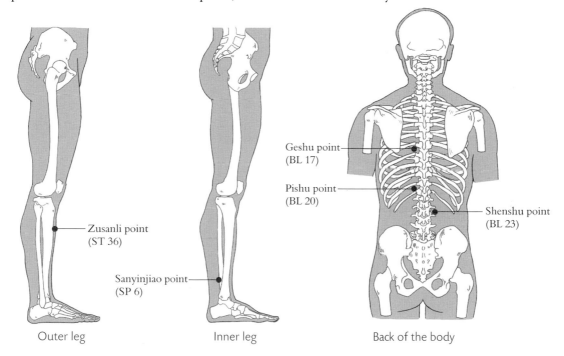

Zusanli point (ST 36)

Sanyinjiao point (SP 6)

Geshu point (BL 17)

Pishu point (BL 20)

Shenshu point (BL 23)

Outer leg   Inner leg   Back of the body

Additional Tips

1. Please choose aerobic exercises of longer duration and lower intensity such as walking, jogging, stair-climbing, dancing or table tennis. You can also do strength exercises with low resistance, such as with small dumbbell. Choose two to three exercises and alternate them according to your personal preference.

2. During exercise, please avoid the hypoglycemic reaction period that may occur after taking medicine. It is best to exercise one hour after meals. You should strive to exercise 30 to 60 minutes, once to twice a day for three to five times a week.

3. Be sure to practice these exercises regularly and follow every step.

4. Stop the exercises under the following circumstances:
- Your blood sugar is not controlled well or is too high.
- Your condition is accompanied by any of various types of acute infection.
- Arrhythmia or angina occurs.
- Urine test reveals obvious increases of red blood cells or protein.
- You experience complications with diabetes including foot problems or lesions.

5. Carry candies or other sugary items so that you can eat them if any symptom of hypoglycemia occurs.

6. When away from home, please carry a card with you, which specifies your name, age, address and telephone, your identity as a diabetes patient, and pertinent information so that others can help you in case of an emergency.

What to Do If You Are Suddenly Attacked by Hypoglycemia during Exercise

Hypoglycemia refers to the excessive decline of blood sugar, resulting in sudden dizziness, blurred vision, nausea and vomiting, abnormal sweating, cold hands and feet, and even fainting. When the blood sugar of diabetes patients fluctuates, especially when undertaking activity not long after the injection and administration of any hypoglycemic agent, hypoglycemia may occur. Some patients can remain in a state of hypoglycemia for a long time due to malnutrition.

If you understand self-help methods and deal with hypoglycemia as soon as it occurs, your symptoms can be relieved rapidly.

1. When a hypoglycemic reaction occurs suddenly, you should first stop exercises. Immediately sit or lie down to ensure blood supply to the head and prevent fainting. If conditions permit, please eat candies at once, or drink about 100 ml of 5%–10% sweet water or sweet beverages. Be sure to keep warm in cold weather, and keep cool and ventilated in hot weather. If your symptoms still cannot be relieved, you need to consult doctors for further diagnosis and treatment, or in severe cases be taken to a hospital, remaining in a horizontal position.

2. In a horizontal position, gently pinch and rub your Hegu point, Shuigou point and Baihui point, one to three minutes for each point. You may need to ask for help from others.

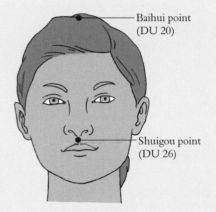

Baihui point (DU 20)

Shuigou point (DU 26)

Front of the head

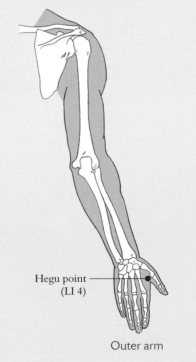

Hegu point (LI 4)

Outer arm

3 | Coronary Heart Disease

Coronary heart disease, also known as coronary atherosclerotic heart disease, is a kind of ischemic heart disease. Although it is the most common disease of the elderly, more and more young people are suffering from this disease. With very complicated causes, coronary heart disease is closely related to age, sex, occupation, nutrition, smoking and drinking habits, stress and other mental influences, heredity and the influence of other diseases.

Patients with typical coronary heart disease would feel chest pain continuously, radiating toward their left shoulder, left back or chest area. However non-typical coronary heart disease is also common, in which sufferers would always only feel outbursts of dull ache in their left chest. There are many degrees of pain, and sometimes there is no obvious ache but only a choking sensation in the chest. Another main symptom is cardiac arrhythmia of various types.

The following introduces self-help methods suitable only for patients with mild coronary heart disease on the basis of systematic treatment.

Meridian and Collateral Exercises

Please spend about 20 minutes every day practicing all sixteen steps of the meridian and collateral exercises in Chapter Two. You can also choose the following steps to practice together or separately, once to twice a day, moderately increasing repetitions over time.

1. Step 3 hand-throwing and tiptoeing: 50 to 100 times, at a low speed and with less amplitude in hand-throwing and less height of tiptoeing. You can make continuous adjustments to this exercise according to your own feelings so that you will not feel uncomfortable in any case.

2. Tapping on and along the spine of Step 14: applying gentle force with your hand and moving up and down the spine for four sequences of four 8-beats

3. Tapping the chest of Step 14: four 8-beats, applying slow and gentle force using a semi-clenched fist

4. Step 15 swaying and shaking: 1 to 2 minutes

5. Step 16 closing eyes meditatively: 1 to 2 minutes

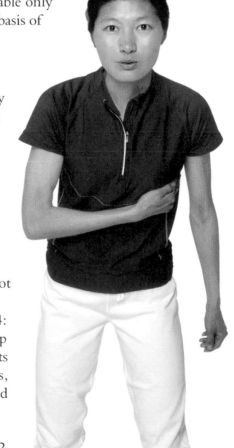

Tapping the chest of Step 14

Self-Massaging

Pinch and rub your Danzhong point, Jiquan point, Hegu point, Neiguan point, Shenmen point, Zhongchong point, Jueyinshu point and Xinshu point. The duration should be for 1 to 2 minutes, once to twice a day when the state of illness is stable. When the state of illness is unstable or aggravated, you can ask others to pinch and rub these points for you while awaiting medical attention.

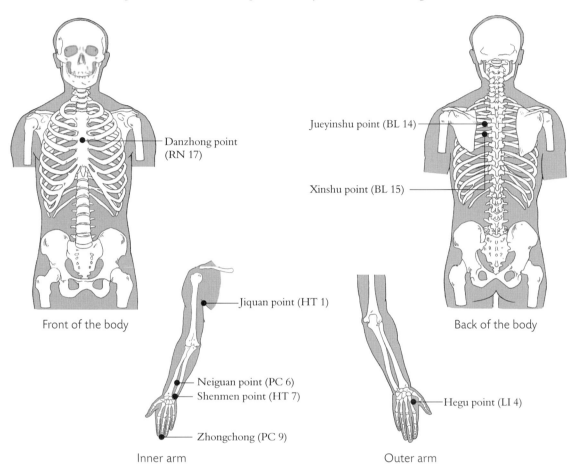

Danzhong point (RN 17)

Front of the body

Jueyinshu point (BL 14)

Xinshu point (BL 15)

Back of the body

Jiquan point (HT 1)

Neiguan point (PC 6)
Shenmen point (HT 7)

Zhongchong (PC 9)

Inner arm

Hegu point (LI 4)

Outer arm

Additional Tips

Patients with coronary heart disease should undertake moderate physical exercise, selecting leisurely activities and controlling the duration within a reasonable scope. Examples of suitable exercises include: strolling, slow dancing, billiards, shuffle board, tai chi, etc. If you experience choking or ache in the chest, palpitation, shortness of breath, abnormal sweating, tachycardia or cardiac arrhythmia during exercise, stop immediately and seek treatment.

In addition patients with coronary heart disease must receive regular medical treatment and observation, maintain an optimistic state of mind, refrain from smoking and drinking, eat a moderate amount of food, and take part in moderate activities, being sure not to overexert themselves.

4 Cervical Degeneration

In recent years, the incidence of cervical degeneration has been higher and higher, and it is increasing affecting younger people, especially office workers and students. People who use computers, sit for work or study, and do not get enough exercise will experience stiff muscles in their neck and back, gradually leading to strain and injury. This can affect the normal physiology of their cervical vertebrae, cause degenerative changes of intervertebral discs and hyperostosis of cervical vertebrae, and eventually lead to cervical degeneration.

Clinically cervical degeneration is usually classified into five types: neck, nerve root, spinal, vertebral artery and sympathic. However, the mixed type predominates.

Patients have different clinical manifestations, but share common symptoms in the early period including: ache in the neck, shoulder and back, dizziness, headache, numbness and weakness in the arms, and muscular atrophy. Since this ailment occurs over time, if attention is paid to daily self-healthcare, it can be easily prevented. In addition if timely treatment and self-adjustment are practiced after symptoms occur, the development of the degeneration may be effectively controlled.

The below-mentioned methods for self treatment are only suitable for patients with mild cervical degeneration.

Meridian and Collateral Exercises

Please spend about 20 minutes every day practicing all sixteen steps of the meridian and collateral exercises in Chapter Two. You can also choose the following steps to practice together or separately, once to twice a day, moderately increasing repetitions over time.

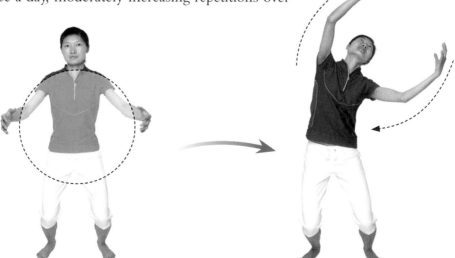

Step 2 holding a "ball" in a horse-riding stance

1. Step 2 holding a "ball" in horse-riding stance: four 8-beats; the amplitude of neck movement can be increased slowly.

2. Neck rotation of Step 6: moving at a low speed and gradually increasing amplitude; four 8-beats

3. Shoulder rotation of Step 6: four 8-beats. When the shoulder rotation ends, stretch your head forward, with your eyes looking upward, and maintain this posture for 5 to 10 seconds.

4. Horizontal neck pulling of Step 10: four 8-beats

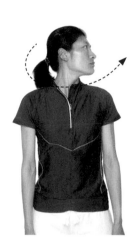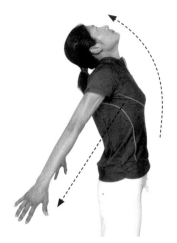

Neck rotation of Step 6

Self-Massaging

Forcefully pinch and rub your Fengchi point, Waiguan point, Dazhui point and Jianjing point for 1 to 2 minutes, once to twice a day. In addition, pinch the muscles of both shoulders and the neck with your palm, which can also relieve your symptoms effectively.

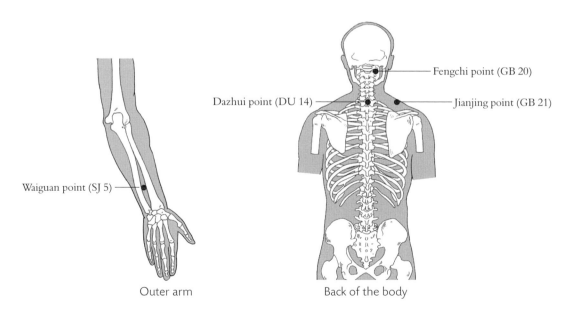

Waiguan point (SJ 5)

Dazhui point (DU 14)

Fengchi point (GB 20)

Jianjing point (GB 21)

Outer arm   Back of the body

Methods for Preventing Cervical Degeneration

1. Select a comfortable, low pillow: About one-third of our life is spent with our head on a pillow so a suitable pillow is vital. A thin pillow stuffed with buckwheat husk is appropriate, and it is best if it is lightly stuffed so that it is convenient to change the shape of the pillow according to body position and feeling.

2. Position your head correctly: While lying on your back, rest your neck on the pillow and compress the buckwheat stuffing with your hand at the part on which the back of your head rests. This will position your head so that it can slightly stretch backward. This state of slight suspension allows the weight of your head to gently pull your cervical vertebrae, which is helpful for maintaining the normal curve. When lying on your side, adjust the stuffing so that the pillow is exactly as thick as your shoulder, eliminating any burden on your neck.

3. Press acupuncture points before sleep: Lie down on your back. Bend your right arm and cushion your neck with your entire palm. Support your left Fengchi point with your middle fingertip. Then pinch your neck forcefully. Pinch and release it immediately, and repeat this action again and again. Then do this on the left and the right side in turn; four 8-beats for each side.

The weight of your head rests on your palms as it moves from side to side when you pinch and release your neck. This is equivalent to using the Zhongchong point to hit the Fengchi point, which produces a very comfortable feeling.

4. Stretch while sitting: During work or study, every half hour you should reach back and embrace the back of chair. If your chair does not have a back, you can shake your hands behind your back. While adding force gradually, withdraw your abdomen and stretch your chest forward. Stretch your head backward and maintain this posture for 20 to 30 seconds. At the same time, slowly rotate your neck from side to side. Next still sit in the chair, cross your arms and tightly hug your shoulders. Forcefully press your shoulders and bend at the waist, keeping your head as close to your legs as possible. Remain still for 10 seconds. Be sure to practice these stretches whenever sitting for long periods of time.

5. Fly kites: This fun activity has many advantages, but it is only suitable for patients with the cervical type of cervical degeneration, and is not necessarily suitable for other types.

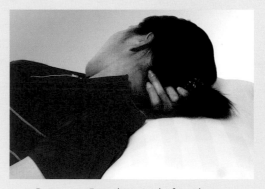

Press your Fengchi point before sleep.

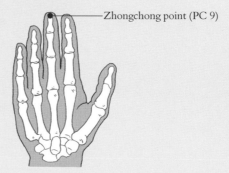

Zhongchong point (PC 9)

Palm

5 Periarthritis of the Shoulders

Periarthritis of the shoulders can be related to the degenerative change of soft tissues around the shoulder joint or to injury. Young people suffer from this disease mostly during physical exercise, and it can result when shoulders are improperly treated after acute or chronic injury. This disease is an aseptic inflammation disease because it is not accompanied by infection.

Main symptoms include ache and limited activity around the shoulder joint. The upper arm may not be able to lift heavy objects or may even become immobile. This is clinically called "frozen shoulder" as the joint seems as if frozen in place due to the degeneration of soft tissue. In addition shoulder ache may also occur, sometimes seriously, sometimes slightly. However it slowly evolves into a continuous ache, which has a definite impact on daily work and life.

Although there is also an acute type, the chronic form is more common. Just as in cervical degeneration, formation is a long-term process. You should give priority to prevention. If you are already suffering from this condition, you should not only receive comprehensive medical treatment but also practice healthcare methods yourself to relieve your symptoms.

Meridian and Collateral Exercises

Please spend about 20 minutes every day practicing all sixteen steps of the meridian and collateral exercises in Chapter Two. You can also choose the following steps to practice together or separately, once to twice a day, moderately increasing repetitions over time.

1. Shoulder rotation of Step 6: slowly for four 8-beats
2. Embrace your head and press your elbows and shoulders of Step 11: slowly for four 8-beats
3. Tapping the area around the Jianyu point and shoulder joint of Step 14: four 8-beats, applying significant force
4. Tapping on and along the spine of Step 14: up and down and back and forth; four times of four 8-beats. Increase gradually, moving upward to the highest point you can reach.

Self-Massaging

Pinch and rub your Yanglao point, Waiguan point, Quchi point, Jianzhen point, Jianyu point and Bingfeng point: 1 to 2 minutes for each point, once to twice a day.

Embrace your head and press your elbows and shoulders of Step 11

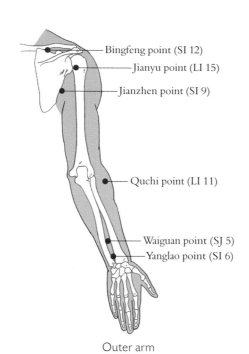

Bingfeng point (SI 12)
Jianyu point (LI 15)
Jianzhen point (SI 9)

Quchi point (LI 11)

Waiguan point (SJ 5)
Yanglao point (SI 6)

Outer arm

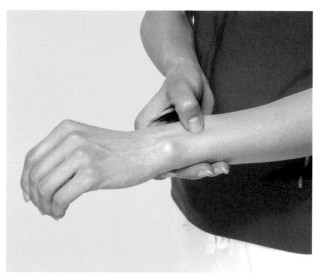

Massage the Waiguan point.

Additional Tips

Patients with periarthritis of the shoulder should keep their shoulder warm, and protect it from wind, cold and humidity, as well as from repeated injury. You can put a moderately hot compress on your shoulder.

Additional Exercise: Climbing the Wall with Your Hands

1. Face the Wall

Efficacy: This is particularly suitable for people who have difficulty raising their arms. The shoulder joint can be stretched in the front and rear direction.

Action: Stand facing the wall, with one arm outstretched in front of you, parallel to the ground. Touch the wall with the fingers facing upward. Gradually climb up the wall with your fingers. At the same time, move your body closer and closer to the wall for four 8-beats until your arm is straight and your entire body touches the wall. Remain still for 5 to 10 seconds, then gradually climb down the wall with

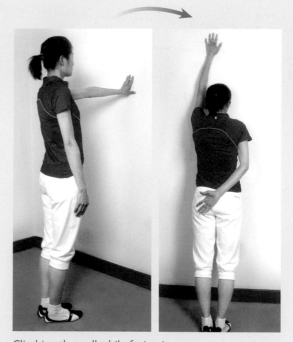

Climbing the wall while facing it

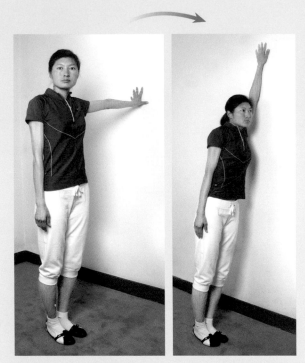

Climbing your fingers while standing perpendicular to the wall

your fingers until you return to your original posture, taking four 8-beats. Practice this on the left and the right side in turn.

2. Stand Perpendicular to the Wall

Efficacy: This action provides sideways stretching of the shoulder joint.

Action: Standing perpendicular to the wall, stretch your arm horizontally toward the wall, touching it with fingers facing upward. Gradually climb up the wall with your fingers, moving your body closer and closer to the wall for four 8-beats. Finally your arm should be straightened with the entire side of your body touching the wall. Remain still for 5 to 10 seconds. Then gradually climb down the wall with your fingers for four 8-beats until you return to your original posture. Practice this on the left and the right side in turn.

3. Press Your Shoulder Against the Wall

Efficacy: This action can help to relax not only the soft tissue around your shoulder but also the muscle groups on the outer side of your chest/abdomen, which are not easily stretched through normal activity.

Action: Stand perpendicular to the wall, bend the arm closest to the wall and place your forearm on your head. Press your elbow into the wall. Then repeatedly squeeze and relax your body against the wall in turn, keeping your body as close to the wall as possible when squeezing. Practice this action slowly for four 8-beats. At the last beat, tightly press your entire body to the wall and remain still for 5 to 10 seconds. Practice this on the left and the right side in turn.

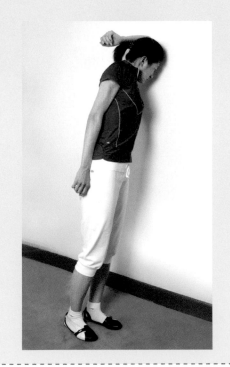

Pressing your shoulder against the wall with bent elbow

6 Lower Back Pain (Backache)

The waist is the hub of the human body, and it is the part of the body most often involved in daily activity and special exercise.

It should be noted that the only lower back pain addressed in this text is that caused by strain of the lumbar muscles and mild osteoarthrosis. Their causes are very similar to those of cervical degeneration and shoulder ache, e.g. retrogression of lumbar vertebrae, acute and chronic athletic injury, long-term exposure to wind, cold and humidity, etc.

Office workers and students often use computers and sit for long periods of time, so that the muscles in their lower back are often in a state of continuous static contraction. This can lead to chronic strain of the lumbar muscles, stasis of qi and blood and weakening of blood circulation, and the development of soft-tissue fascia with pain due to such various nodules. At this time, the patient can often feel these nodules of fibrosis in the lower back.

This kind of lower back pain is often accompanied by waist stiffness, limited movement, obvious decline of flexibility, and sometimes ache or numbness in the hip and outer side of the lower limbs.

If this condition has already developed, you should not only receive comprehensive treatment, but also incorporate the following methods to take action to relieve your symptoms.

Meridian and Collateral Exercises

Please spend about 20 minutes every day practicing all sixteen steps of the meridian and collateral exercises in Chapter Two. You can also choose the following steps to practice together or separately, once to twice a day, moderately increasing repetitions over time.

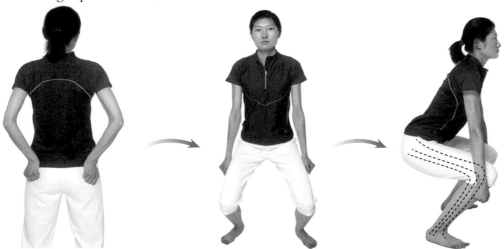

Tapping the buttocks and the outer thigh and calf of Step 14

1. Step 2 holding a "ball" in a horse-riding stance: slowly for four 8-beats

2. Waist rotation of Step 6: slowly for four 8-beats. You can press the relevant acupuncture points or pain points at your waist with your fists, thus enhancing the effect through simultaneous massage.

3. Tapping the Qihai point and Mingmen point of Step 14: four 8-beats, applying more force with your hand

4. Tapping the buttocks and the outer thigh and calf of Step 14: four 8-beats, applying more force with your hand

5. Tapping on and along the spine of Step 14: up and down and back and forth for four times of four 8-beats

Self-Massaging

Pinch and rub your Mingmen point, Shenshu point, Qihaishu point, Yaoyangguan point, Huantiao point and Weizhong point: 1 to 2 minutes for each point, once to twice a day.

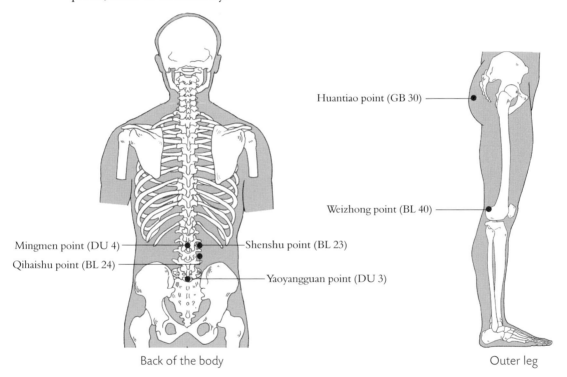

Back of the body   Outer leg

Additional Tips

People with ache in the waist or lower back need to keep these areas warm, and protect them from wind, cold and humidity. They may choose to use a hot compress on these areas in moderation.

Sitting posture is very important. Whenever seated, including in an office, classroom, restaurant or vehicle, you should try to tightly press the lumbosacral region into the back of the seat, which can obviously relieve pressure and prevent pain.

Additional Exercise: Stretching of the Lumbar Muscles

1. Back Flying

Lie on your stomach on a mat or bed. Place your arms alongside your body or stretch them forward alongside your head. Raise your arms and legs at the same time. Using the force of your lumbar and dorsal muscles, gradually raise your body for a count of one 8-beat to four 8-beats, or complete this lifting action several times, taking a short rest in the middle.

2. Waist Suspension

Lie face down, with your upper chest on a bed or chair, and your lower legs (from the knees) on a chair or stool. Your waist should be suspended in the air, with your body straight and parallel to the ground. Remain like this for one to five minutes. If this becomes easy, you can gradually add objects, e.g. a sandbag, to your waist to further reinforce your lumbar muscles.

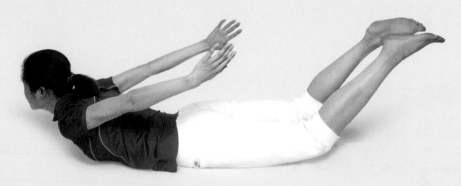

Back flying

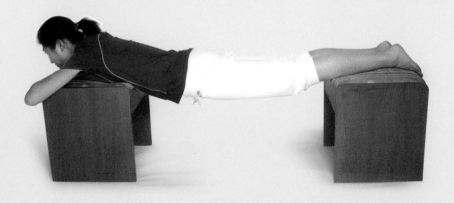

Suspend your waist in the air.

7 | Knee Pain

There are many causes of knee pain, with the most common being arthritis, trauma and long-time exposure to adverse environmental conditions. The knee pain caused by trauma is mostly acute, and in that case requires immediate medical treatment. The treatment proposed here is only for knee pain caused by osteoarthritis.

Pain in the knee joint can be caused by strain or retrogression. Its main symptoms include pain, swelling, deformity and activity limitation. After a good rest, the pain will usually lessen.

In the case of patella and cartilage injury, typical manifestations include: more pain when going downstairs than when going upstairs; more pain when squatting; different degrees of swelling; long-term ache; obvious atrophy of quadriceps femoris; decline of flexibility of the knee joint; clearly evident stiffness; occasional weakness or locking when walking; and a flipping or rubbing sound from the knee joint.

Since this condition develops slowly, it is best to use self-treatment methods to relieve the symptoms. Even patients with serious symptoms should practice moderate functional training, which is different from ordinary exercise. These methods are also suitable for other injuries that cause knee pain, and they can be used during the recovery period as a means of auxiliary treatment.

Meridian and Collateral Exercises

Please spend about 20 minutes every day practicing all sixteen steps of the meridian and collateral exercises in Chapter Two. You can also choose the following steps to practice together or separately, once to twice a day, moderately increasing repetitions over time.

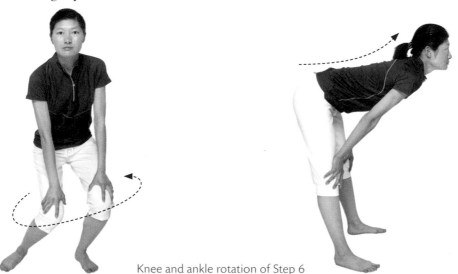

Knee and ankle rotation of Step 6

1. Step 2 holding a "ball" in a horse-riding stance: using a more shallow squat if necessary; four 8-beats
2. Knee and ankle rotation of Step 6: four 8-beats, slowly
3. Tapping the buttocks and the outer thigh and calf of Step 14: four 8-beats respectively, applying more force with your hand
4. Tapping the inside of the thigh and calf of Step 14: four 8-beats respectively, applying more force with your hand
5. Step 12 letting go and taking in breath: using a shallower squat if necessary; four 8-beats

Self-Massaging

Pinch and rub your Yinlingquan point, Yanglingquan point, Weizhong point and Liangqiu point: 1 to 2 minutes for each point, once to twice a day.

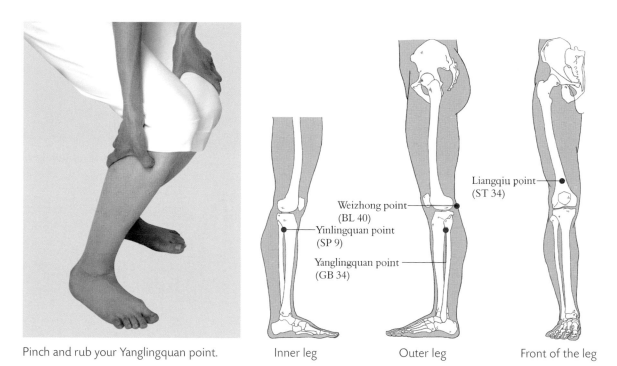

Pinch and rub your Yanglingquan point.

Inner leg   Outer leg   Front of the leg

Additional Tips

Please keep your knee joint warm, and protect it from wind, cold and humidity. You can use moderately hot compress on your knee.

Avoid over-using your knee, especially avoiding exercises that obviously abrade your articular cartilage. These include frequent squatting and rising; leaping; mountain-climbing; some forms of tai chi (low-position); and activities involving an excessively high speed. However you can bend and stretch your knee in a sitting or reclining posture, act as if pedaling a "bicycle," raise your straightened leg with a light load, and engage in any other functional training.

Additional Exercise: Horse-Riding Stance

The horse-riding stance is almost essential for preventing injuries of the knee joint and during recovery. Some people fear that this stance can aggravate knee problems. This is not the case, as the stance is only a static exercise.

The contraction of the strong muscles of the thigh can greatly improve the blood circulation of knee joint. Moreover the contraction of this muscle group will not produce movement of the knee, and can prevent new abrasion to the inner and outer tissues of the knee joint.

If the knee pain is from a new injury to the cartilage, ligament and synovium of meniscus and articular surface caused in the process of exercise, the horse-riding stance can also be practiced. It can strengthen the quadriceps femoris, reinforce the stability of the knee joint, increase the blood supply to the knee and promote metabolism, regeneration and restoration of injured tissues. This will reinforce the knee's resistance to further injuries and accelerate recovery.

Therefore this stance is recommended for most athletes, helping to prevent athletic injury and promote recovery. Patients with knee osteoarthritis and those with other chronic knee pain can also practice the horse-riding stance every day. There are two specific methods.

1. Natural Horse-Riding Stance
Stand up straight, and separate your legs so that they are wider than your shoulders.

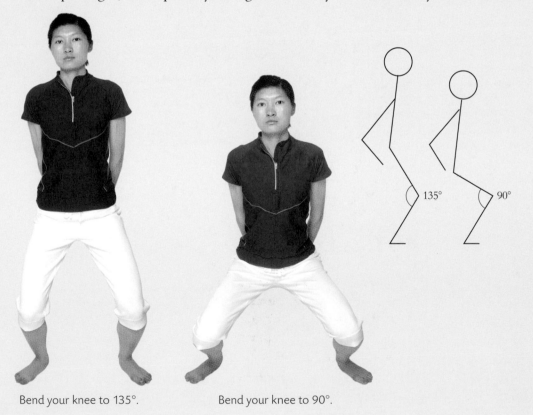

Bend your knee to 135°.   Bend your knee to 90°.

Stretch your chest forward and pull in your abdomen. Clasp your hands in front of your chest or behind your back. Squat down, starting off gently at the beginning, and bend so as to make an angle of about 135° from the floor. As your knee joint and quadriceps femoris allow, gradually sink down, moving to an angle of 90°. This is difficult, so if you cannot reach this angle just bend less deeply.

The duration of this stance can be slowly extended. It is best to practice it four times at a stretch, with each squat lasting for 1 minute. You can eventually extend to 3 to 5 minutes, with a rest of 1 minute. Remember to tap and relax the front of your thigh for 1 to 2 minutes after the practice.

2. Horse-Riding Stance Against a Wall

Against expectation, it is more difficult to maintain a horse-riding stance against the wall than it is to maintain a natural horse-riding stance.

During the natural stance, when your quadriceps femoris begin to fatigue, your body will naturally move forward and backward, changing the load-carrying center of gravity so that different muscle fibers can rest in turn. This lessens stress on the entire muscle group. Moreover since the line of your center of gravity does not always run through your knee joint, the improvement of blood circulation is also influenced.

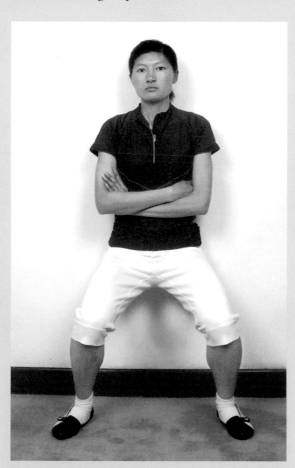

In addition a natural horse-riding stance produces a protective action of reducing intensity as matter of course. Your body gradually leans forward and your lumbar muscles provide assistance, resulting in decrease of the recuperative effect for your knee joint. Moreover this may also strain your lumbar muscles. Therefore the method of maintaining a horse-riding stance against the wall is preferable, as the stance retains all its benefits while the defects of the natural stance are eliminated.

Regarding the practice in this stance, you can follow the directions regarding the angle of the knee bend, the duration and repetitions outlined in the section of "natural horse-riding stance."

Horse-riding stance against a wall

8 Shoulder and Back Pain

There are many causes of shoulder and back pain; here we will only discuss those caused by myofascitis of the shoulder and back.

Many occurrences of shoulder and back pain have causes similar to those of cervical degeneration: long-term exposure to wind, cold, humidity; injury; and long-term use of computers or sedentary work or study. In particular pain can occur when at the computer, with only the wrists on the desk top and both arms are suspended in air for a long time. The chronic strain of shoulder and back muscles, qi and blood stasis, and weakening of blood circulation lead to the circular nodules, strip-like nodules and other fibrotic lesions occurring to soft tissues. Pain can result from aseptic inflammation of muscle and fascia.

An obvious characteristic of this type of pain is that these nodules can be felt at the shoulder and back. Please note that ache of the shoulder and back often exists at the same time as cervical degeneration. Treating yourself through the following methods can help to relieve the condition and the pain.

Meridian and Collateral Exercises

Please spend about 20 minutes every day practicing all sixteen steps of the meridian and collateral exercises in Chapter Two. You can also choose the following steps to practice together or separately, once to twice a day, moderately increasing repetitions over time.

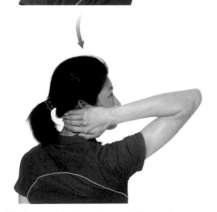

1. Shoulder rotation of Step 6: four 8-beats; slowly with the amplitude gradually increasing

2. Horizontal neck pulling of Step 10: four 8-beats, slowly, and applying more force

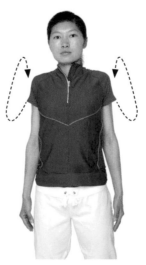
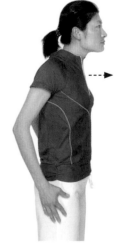

Horizontal neck pulling of Step 10

Shoulder rotation of Step 6

3. Embrace your head and press your elbows and shoulders of Step 11: four 8-beats, slowly

4. Tapping the area around the Jianyu point and shoulder joint of Step 14: four 8-beats, applying more force

5. Tapping the Tianzong point of Step 14: four 8-beats, applying more force

6. Tapping the Jianjing point and Bingfeng point of Step 14: four 8-beats, applying more force

7. Tapping on and along the spine of Step 14: up and down and back and forth for four times of four 8-beats; increase gradually to the highest point you can reach

Self-Massaging

Pinch and rub your Dazhui point, Tianzong point, Jianjing point and Bingfeng point: 1 to 2 minutes for each point, once to twice a day.

Additional Tips

Please keep your shoulders and back warm, protect them from the environment, and use a moderate hot compress on them.

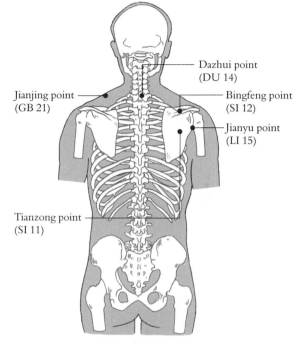

Dazhui point (DU 14)

Jianjing point (GB 21)

Bingfeng point (SI 12)

Jianyu point (LI 15)

Tianzong point (SI 11)

Back of the body

Additional Exercise: Hug Your Shoulders Tightly

During work or study, about every half hour, you should strongly hug your shoulders. First sit straight on a chair, with your legs extended in front of you. Cross your arms at your chest and grasp your shoulders with opposite hands. Lower your head and bend at the waist, moving your body toward your legs. Maintain this posture for 10 seconds, and then expand your chest forcefully for 8 beats.

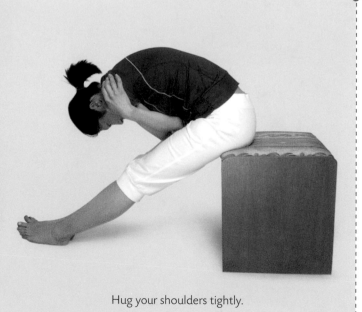

Hug your shoulders tightly.

9 Headache

Headache can be a reaction caused by the disorder of the regulatory function of blood vessel nerves or the symptom of some diseases. While headaches discussed here do not include those caused by various organic diseases, I will focus on functional headaches of the blood vessel nerve. In this case the attack is mostly manifested as migraine, and sometimes nerve headaches can also be manifested as pain in two sides and the top of head. Applying self-healthcare methods during treatment can also help to relieve symptoms and ache.

Meridian and Collateral Exercises

Please spend about 20 minutes every day practicing all sixteen steps of the meridian and collateral exercises in Chapter Two. You can also choose the following steps to practice together or separately, once to twice a day, moderately increasing repetitions over time.

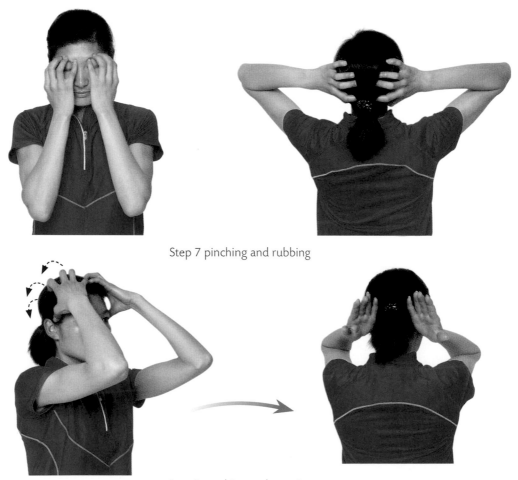

Step 7 pinching and rubbing

Step 8 combing and scraping

1. Step 7 pinching and rubbing: four times of four 8-beats, applying more force

2. Step 8 combing and scraping: two times of four 8-beats, applying more force

3. Step 15 swaying and shaking: 2 to 3 minutes

4. Step 16 closing eyes meditatively: 2 to 3 minutes

Self-Massaging

You can choose either of the following two groups, or practice them in turn. Pinch and rub each point for 1 to 2 minutes, once to twice a day.

1. Taichong point, Fenglong point, Taiyang point, Cuanzhu point, Shangxing point and Touwei point

2. Yongquan point, Baihui point, Yintang point, Sizhukong point and Fengchi point

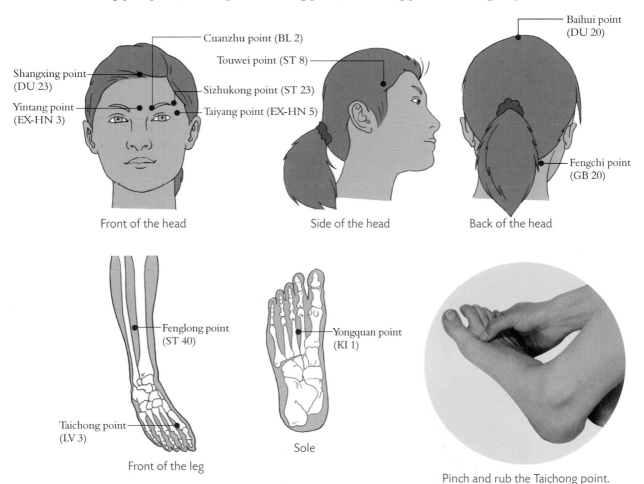

Cuanzhu point (BL 2)
Touwei point (ST 8)
Shangxing point (DU 23)
Sizhukong point (ST 23)
Yintang point (EX-HN 3)
Taiyang point (EX-HN 5)
Baihui point (DU 20)
Fengchi point (GB 20)

Front of the head   Side of the head   Back of the head

Fenglong point (ST 40)
Yongquan point (KI 1)
Taichong point (LV 3)

Front of the leg   Sole

Pinch and rub the Taichong point.

Additional Tips

When you have a headache, you need to relax yourself, maintain a good mood, drink tea, enjoy light music, watch comic programs, etc. You should refrain from smoking, and avoid noise or disturbances.

10 | Common Cold

Colds occur frequently, and I will only discuss the common cold in the following. When the common cold is accompanied by bacterial infection, you can consider using some antibacterial agents for treatment. Otherwise, I strongly suggest relying on your own immunological competence for recovery. At the onset of a common cold, using the following methods may allow you to recover without medicine.

Meridian and Collateral Exercises

Please spend about 20 minutes every day practicing all sixteen steps of the meridian and collateral exercises in Chapter Two. You can also choose the following steps to practice together or separately, once to twice a day, moderately increasing repetitions over time.

1. Step 7 pinching and rubbing: four times of four 8-beats, applying more force

2. Step 8 combing and scraping: twice of four 8-beats, applying more force

3. Push and rub your face of Step 9: twice of four 8-beats, applying more force

4. Tapping the Feishu point and Dazhui point of Step 14: four 8-beats, applying more force

5. Tapping on and along the spine of Step 14: up and down and back and forth, four times of four 8-beats

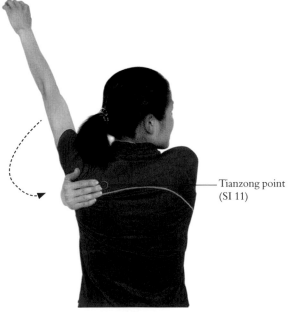

Tianzong point
(SI 11)

Tap your Tianzong point.

Recommendations of Life Style

Be sure to wash your face, rinse your mouth and soak your nose with cold water in the early morning all year round. While taking a shower, it is recommended to use cold and hot water in turn, to increase your body's adaptability.

Other recommendations include drinking more water and refraining from smoking. Keep yourself warm and adapt your clothing along with changes of air temperature. When caught in the rain or exposed to any other wind or cold, drink a glass of boiled water with ginger and sugar as soon as possible.

Self-Massaging

1. To treat common cold: Massage according to your symptoms. Pinch and rub selected points for 2 to 3 minutes; you can also do it repeatedly.
- Headache: Taiyang point, Fengchi point
- Stuffy nose: Yingxiang point
- Fever: Hegu point, Quchi point
- Cough: Feishu point, Danzhong point
- Sore throat: Tiantu point

2. To prevent common cold: You can choose the Zusanli point, Hegu point and Neiguan point. Gently pinch and rub each point for 1 to 2 minutes. During times when colds occur frequently, pinch and rub once to twice a day.

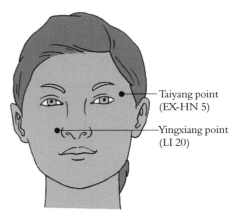

Taiyang point (EX-HN 5)

Yingxiang point (LI 20)

Front of the head

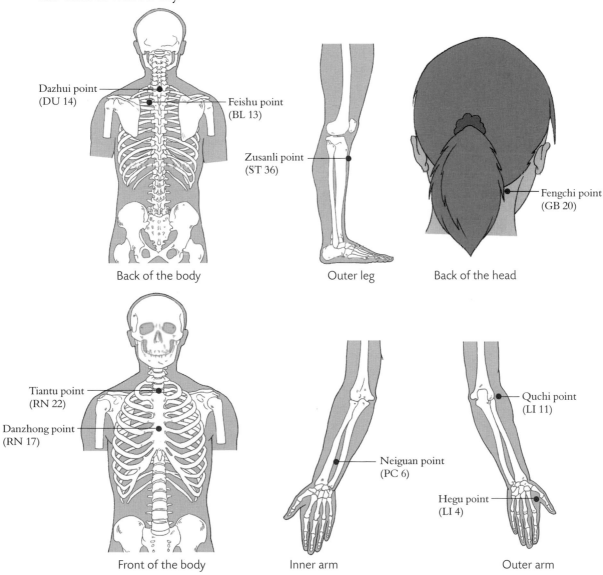

Dazhui point (DU 14)

Feishu point (BL 13)

Zusanli point (ST 36)

Fengchi point (GB 20)

Back of the body

Outer leg

Back of the head

Tiantu point (RN 22)

Danzhong point (RN 17)

Neiguan point (PC 6)

Quchi point (LI 11)

Hegu point (LI 4)

Front of the body

Inner arm

Outer arm

11 | Cough

The cough is the most common symptom among diseases of the respiratory system. It is a protective reaction that expels foreign matter in the respiratory tract out of the body, maintaining the integrity of the respiratory tract and ensuring smooth respiration.

However violent coughing produces a negative effect on the body. For example the drastic rise of pressure in the chest and abdomen and the strong contraction of muscles can cause the rupture of small blood vessels and internal hemorrhage, increase the burden on the heart, cause fluctuation of blood pressure, and, therefore, bring about many potential risks.

Generally speaking, mild coughing does not require treatment. However serious coughing should not only be treated with cough-suppressants, but should also be treated with expectorant or anti-inflammatory drugs at the same time.

What I will introduce lays particular emphasis on the following point: When undertaking treatment of diseases that cause coughing, you should use self-healthcare methods to help relieve your symptoms, increase physical resistance and promote recovery.

Meridian and Collateral Exercises

Please spend about 20 minutes every day practicing all sixteen steps of the meridian and collateral exercises in Chapter Two. You can also choose the following steps to practice together or separately, once to twice a day, moderately increasing repetitions over time.

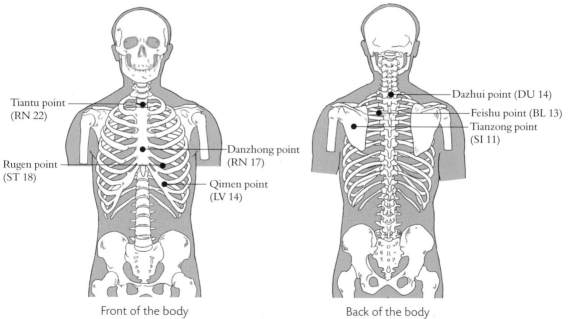

Tiantu point (RN 22)

Rugen point (ST 18)

Danzhong point (RN 17)

Qimen point (LV 14)

Dazhui point (DU 14)

Feishu point (BL 13)

Tianzong point (SI 11)

Front of the body

Back of the body

1. Tapping the Feishu point and Dazhui point of Step 14: four 8-beats
2. Tapping the Tianzong point of Step 14: four 8-beats
3. Tapping the chest of Step 14: four 8-beats, gently

Self-Massaging

Pinch and rub your Qimen point, Rugen point, Danzhong point, Tiantu point, Dazhui point, Feishu point, and Tianzong point. Pinch and rub each point for 1 to 2 minutes, several times a day.

Additional Tips

To maintain respiratory health, it is helpful to walk and breathe deeply in parks, woods or greenbelts. In addition, you must refrain from smoking, which is very important for patients of chronic cough.

12 | Stomachache

There are many causes of stomachache, which can be roughly classified into pathological changes or dysfunction of the stomach.

Cases of the latter (e.g. spastic pain of the stomach caused by exposure to wind/cold; raw, pungent and cold foods; and excited mood) can be relieved with self-healthcare methods.

For stomachache with pathological changes, please first receive medical diagnosis and treatment. During treatment, you can also try these methods to aid the therapy and relieve your pain.

Meridian and Collateral Exercises

Please spend about 20 minutes every day practicing all sixteen steps of the meridian and collateral exercises in Chapter Two. You can also choose the following steps to practice together or separately, once to twice a day, moderately increasing repetitions over time.

1. Waist rotation of Step 6: four 8-beats. While rotating clench your hands into fists and place them on your waist and back, supporting your Pishu point and Weishu point with your finger joints.

2. Push and rub your chest and abdomen of Step 9: four 8-beats, exerting more force

3. Tapping the Qihai point and Mingmen point of Step 14: four 8-beats, exerting more force

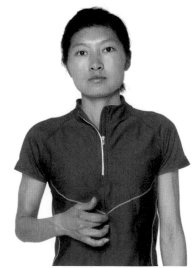

Pinch and rub your Shangwan point.

4. Tapping the outer thigh and calf of Step 14: four 8-beats, exerting more force to tap the Zusanli point and Fenglong point

5. Tapping on and along the spine of Step 14: up and down and back and forth for four times of four 8-beats, exerting more force

Self-Massaging

Pinch and rub your Shangwan point, Zhongwan point, Neiguan point, Weishu point, Weicang point and Zusanli point. 1 to 2 minutes for each point, several times a day.

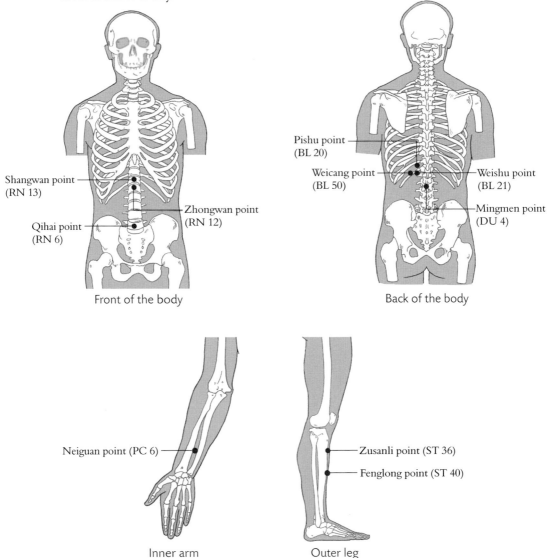

Pishu point
(BL 20)

Weicang point
(BL 50)

Weishu point
(BL 21)

Mingmen point
(DU 4)

Shangwan point
(RN 13)

Zhongwan point
(RN 12)

Qihai point
(RN 6)

Front of the body

Back of the body

Neiguan point (PC 6)

Zusanli point (ST 36)

Fenglong point (ST 40)

Inner arm

Outer leg

Additional Tips

Protect your stomach from exposure to wind/cold; avoid drinking or eating raw, pungent or cold food; and use a moderate hot compress on your stomach. It is also helpful to regulate your mood and maintain an optimistic outlook.

13   Gastroptosis

Gastroptosis is the abnormal downward displacement of the stomach. It is defined by a state wherein the lower edge of the stomach reaches the pelvic cavity when the patient is in a standing position; a B-ultrasound test is usually needed for a definite diagnosis.

Gastroptosis is directly caused by the slackness and subsidence of tissues that are suspended around the stomach and hold it in place. For example, deficient suspension force of the diaphragm; flaccidity of liver-stomach and diaphragm-stomach ligaments and abdominal muscles; and problems with physical development lead to weakening tension of the stomach.

Patients with mild gastroptosis generally have no symptoms. Those suffering from obvious gastroptosis have such symptoms as lack of appetite, constipation, noticeable discomfort in the upper stomach after meals, full stomach, dull pain, nausea and belching. After too much standing or exertion, symptoms are aggravated. Untimely treatment may bring about emaciation, weakness, palpitation and insomnia.

The following self-healthcare methods are only applicable to patients with mild gastroptosis as an adjuvant therapy.

Meridian and Collateral Exercises

Please spend about 20 minutes every day practicing all sixteen steps of the meridian and collateral exercises in Chapter Two. You can also choose the following steps to practice together or separately, once to twice a day, moderately increasing repetitions over time.

1. Waist rotation of Step 6: four 8-beats. While rotating place your fists on your lower back. Support your Pishu point and Weishu point with the joints in

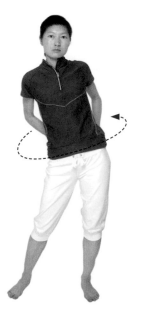
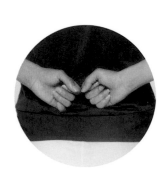
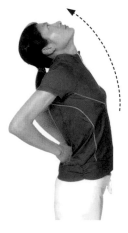

Waist rotation of Step 6

your finger and your palms so they can continuously massage your acupuncture points.

2. Tapping the Qihai point and Mingmen point of Step 14: four 8-beats, applying gentle force with your hand

3. Tapping the outer thigh and calf of Step 14: four 8-beats. Tap your Zusanli point and Fenglong point more frequently, applying a moderate force with your hand

4. Step 13 pushing a "wall": from a high position, four 8-beats

5. Tapping on and along the spine of Step 14: up and down and back and forth; four times of four 8-beats, applying gentle force with your hand

Self-Massaging

Pinch and rub your Qihai point, Zhongwan point, Weishu point, Pishu point, Zusanli point and Neiguan point. 1 to 3 minutes for each point, once to twice a day.

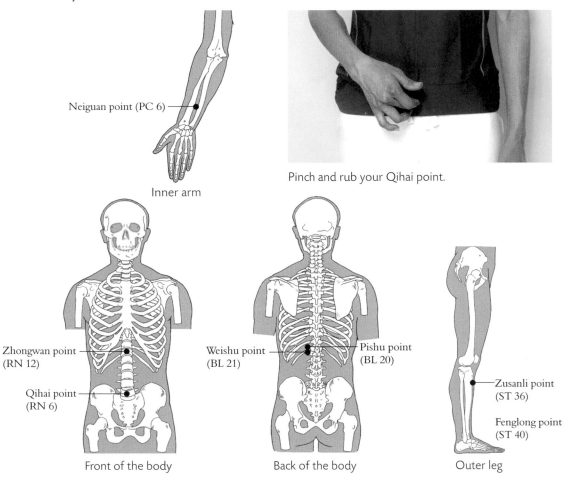

Neiguan point (PC 6)

Inner arm

Pinch and rub your Qihai point.

Zhongwan point (RN 12)

Qihai point (RN 6)

Front of the body

Weishu point (BL 21)

Pishu point (BL 20)

Back of the body

Zusanli point (ST 36)

Fenglong point (ST 40)

Outer leg

Additional Tips

Do not take in too much food. It is also better not to exercise immediately after eating, or to exercise too strenuously at any time.

14 Fatty Liver

Taking in too much food or increasing the content of fat, as well as poor nutrition, can make fat accumulate in the liver through the catabolism of fat metabolism. This results in fatty liver, which can be discovered and diagnosed through such tests as B-ultrasound.

Mild fatty liver may have no symptoms. During its gradual development, such reactions as loss of appetite, lack of strength, abdominal distension, and hepatic region discomfort or dull pain may occur. Along with the aggravation of fatty liver, liver cirrhosis may emerge and other symptoms including nausea and vomiting may also occur.

Patients with mild fatty liver can practice some of the following methods as an auxiliary therapy.

Meridian and Collateral Exercises

Please spend about 20 minutes every day practicing all sixteen steps of the meridian and collateral exercises in Chapter Two. You can also choose the following steps to practice together or separately, once to twice a day, moderately increasing repetitions over time.

1. Waist rotation of Step 6: four 8-beats. While rotating place your fists at your waist and back, and support your Ganshu point and Danshu point with the joints of your fingers and your palms so that they can be massaged continuously.

2. Push and rub your chest and abdomen of Step 9: four 8-beats, exerting a moderate force with your hand

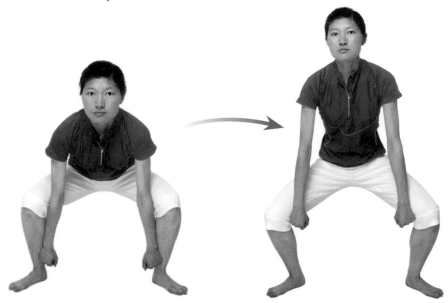

Tapping the inside of the thigh and calf of Step 14

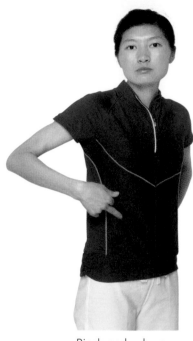

Pinch and rub your
Zhangmen point.

3. Tapping the Qihai point and Mingmen point of Step 14: four 8-beats, exerting a moderate force with your hand

4. Tapping the inside of the thigh and calf of Step 14: four 8-beats, patting the Sanyinjiao point more frequently

5. Step 13 pushing a "wall": from a high position for four 8-beats

6. Tapping on and along the spine of Step 14: up and down and back and forth; four times of four 8-beats, exerting a moderate force with your hand

Self-Massaging

Pinch and rub your Dabao point, Qimen point, Shangwan point, Zhangmen point, Zusanli point and Sanyinjiao point. Exert force counterclockwise for 1 to 3 minutes, once to twice a day.

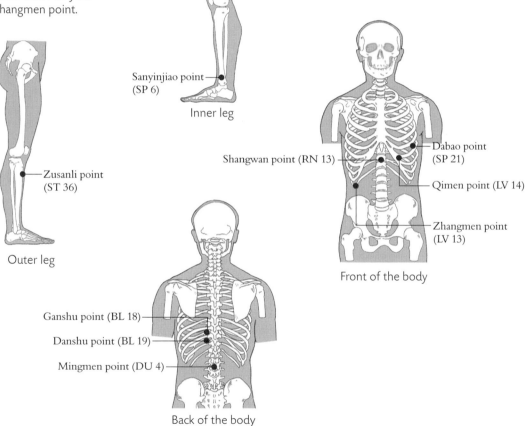

Sanyinjiao point (SP 6)

Inner leg

Zusanli point (ST 36)

Outer leg

Shangwan point (RN 13)

Dabao point (SP 21)

Qimen point (LV 14)

Zhangmen point (LV 13)

Front of the body

Ganshu point (BL 18)

Danshu point (BL 19)

Mingmen point (DU 4)

Back of the body

Additional Tips

Patients with fatty liver should refrain from drinking alcohol and abide by a balanced diet, including eating fewer desserts and refraining from snacks.

15 | Diarrhea

As a common symptom of diseases of the digestive system, diarrhea has many causes. Here I only introduce the simple diarrhea caused by gastrointestinal dysfunction attributed to cold, as defined by TCM. This kind of diarrhea is caused by a disorder of the relaxing and contracting functions of the smooth muscle of the gastrointestinal tract. It is not caused by the infection of microorganisms, and therefore antibiotics are not recommended, but you can practice the following methods for treatment.

Meridian and Collateral Exercises

Please spend about 20 minutes every day practicing all sixteen steps of the meridian and collateral exercises in Chapter Two. You can also choose the following steps to practice together or separately, once to twice a day, moderately increasing repetitions over time.

1. Push and rub your abdomen of Step 9: overlapping your palms, gently push and rub your abdomen counterclockwise for 100 to 200 circles

2. Tapping the Qihai point and Mingmen point of Step 14: four 8-beats, tapping gently with your hand

3. Tapping on and along the spine of Step 14: up and down and back and forth for four times of four 8-beats, exerting gentle force with your hand

Self-Massaging

Gently rub your Zhongwan point, Shenque point, Tianshu point, Qihai point, Guanyuan point and Zusanli point clockwise for 1 to 3 minutes, once to twice a day.

Press your Tianshu point.

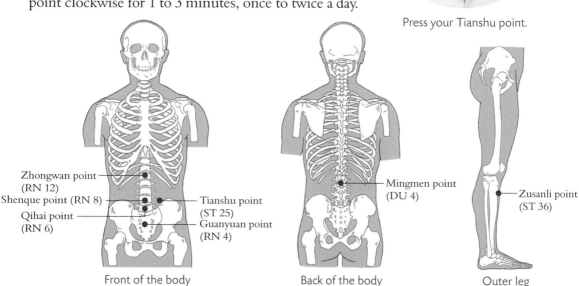

Zhongwan point (RN 12)
Shenque point (RN 8)
Qihai point (RN 6)
Tianshu point (ST 25)
Guanyuan point (RN 4)
Mingmen point (DU 4)
Zusanli point (ST 36)

Front of the body

Back of the body

Outer leg

Additional Tips

1. Fast for one day: Only drink sweet saline water; 200 to 300 ml each time for a total amount of 1,500 to 2,500 ml. If you must eat something, try some noodles or porridge.

2. Moxibustion: This is a very effective therapy for stopping diarrhea. Suspending a mugwort stick at your navel (Shenque point) for 5 to 10 minutes can sometimes produce the desired effect immediately. Ordinary spastic stomachache can also be relieved with this method.

16 Vaginitis

Vaginitis is the inflammation of the vaginal mucous membrane and the connective tissue underneath. It is a common disease, and its main clinical characteristics are a change of the character of leucorrhea (discharge) and itching and burning pain of the vulva. Dyspareunia, or painful intercourse, is also common. When the infection involves the urethral canal such symptoms as painful or urgent urination will occur.

Common vaginitis includes the following types: bacterial vaginitis, trichomonas vaginitis, monilial or mycotic vaginitis and senile vaginitis. While systematic gynecological treatment is necessary, self-healthcare methods can also be used for adjuvant therapy.

Meridian and Collateral Exercises

Please spend about 20 minutes every day practicing all sixteen steps of the meridian and collateral exercises in Chapter Two. You can also choose the following steps to practice together or separately, once to twice a day, moderately increasing repetitions over time.

1. Waist rotation of Step 6: four 8-beats. While rotating your waist, always place your fists at your waist and back. Support your Guanyuanshu point and various sacrum points (Baliao points) with the joints of your fingers and your palms so that they can be massaged continuously.

2. Hip rotation of Step 6: four 8-beats

3. Tapping the inside of the thigh and calf of Step 14: four 8-beats; tapping the Sanyinjiao point more frequently and applying moderate force with your hand

4. Tapping on and along the spine of Step 14: up and down and back and forth for four times of four 8-beats, applying moderate force with your hand

Self-Massaging

Pinch and rub your Yinbai point, Xingjian point, Taichong point, Jimai point and Huiyin point. 1 to 2 minutes for each point, once to twice a day.

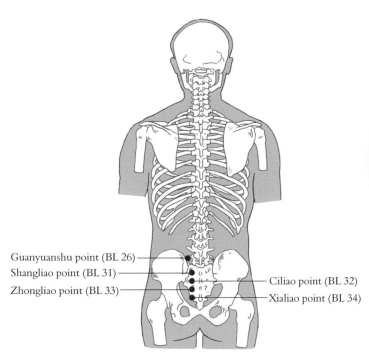

Guanyuanshu point (BL 26)
Shangliao point (BL 31)
Zhongliao point (BL 33)
Ciliao point (BL 32)
Xialiao point (BL 34)

Back of the body

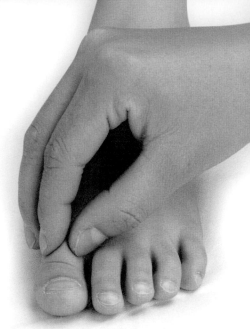

Pinch and rub your Xingjian point.

Additional Tips

Pay attention to personal hygiene. Choose underwear with good air permeability, and do not wear trousers that are too tight.

Moderately increase various exercises of the abdominal muscles, including lifting of the groin region 50 to 100 times before sleep.

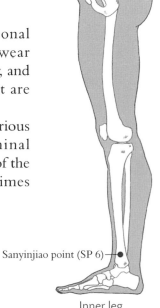

Sanyinjiao point (SP 6)

Inner leg

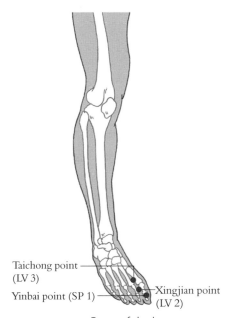

Taichong point (LV 3)
Yinbai point (SP 1)
Xingjian point (LV 2)

Front of the leg

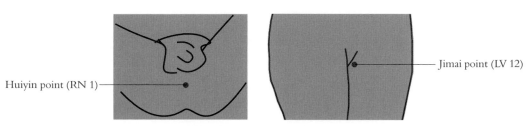

Huiyin point (RN 1)

Jimai point (LV 12)

Front of the body, pelvic region

17 Menstrual Disorder and Pelvic Inflammation

Menstrual disorder is manifested as irregular menstruation or such symptoms as stomachache, mood fluctuations and nerve dysfunction.

There are many causes of menstrual disorder, which fall under pathological or functional disorder. Pathological disorder is usually caused by secondary diseases, including diseases of the genital system (infection, ovarian tumor, myoma of the uterus, hydatid mole, ectopic pregnancy) and systemic diseases (hypertension, diabetes, blood disease, endocrinopathy). These need timely and systematic medical treatment.

Functional menstrual disorder is usually related to such factors as mental or physical overwork, exposure to stimulation of wind/cold and humidity, dysfunction of vegetative nerves, insanity, and nutritional disorders caused by excessive dieting. The following only applies to methods for treating functional menstrual disorder.

Female internal genitalia are surrounded, fixed and protected by connective tissues within the pelvic cavity. The infection of these tissues is called pelvic inflammation, which is a common female disease. Acute pelvic inflammation should be treated medically as soon as possible.

Chronic pelvic inflammation is often caused by non-radical treatment of acute pelvic inflammation, or the overall poor health of patients and the delay of the course of disease. The symptoms include: swelling pain of the lower abdomen, lumbosacral ache, increased leucorrhea and increased menses. Patients may also experience more serious reactions during the menstrual period, fatigue, low-grade fever and insomnia.

On the basis of continuous systematic treatment, self-healthcare methods can be used to reinforce resistance, improve overall body condition, and help relieve symptoms.

Meridian and Collateral Exercises

Please spend about 20 minutes every day practicing all sixteen steps of the meridian and collateral exercises in Chapter Two. You can also choose the following steps to practice together or separately, once to twice a day, moderately increasing repetitions over time.

1. Waist rotation of Step 6: four 8-beats. While rotating always place your fists at your waist and back, and support your Guanyuanshu point and various sacrum holes (Baliao points) with the joints of your fingers and your palms so they can be massaged continuously.

2. Hip rotation of Step 6: four 8-beats

3. Ear-lifting of Step 10: two 8-beats each on the left and right

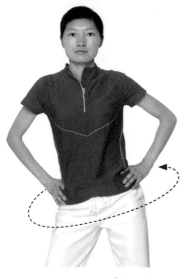
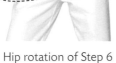

Hip rotation of Step 6

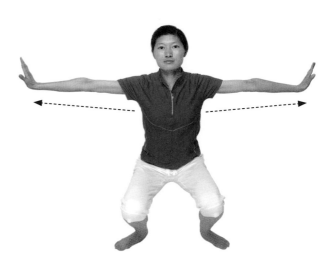

Step 13 pushing a "wall"

4. Push and rub your chest and abdomen of Step 9: four 8-beats, applying moderate force with your hand

5. Tapping the Qihai point and Mingmen point of Step 14: four 8-beats, exerting moderate force with your hand

6. Step 13 pushing a "wall": from a high position for four 8-beats, gradually transitioning to full squat and rise

7. Tapping on and along the spine of Step 14: up and down and back and forth for four times of four 8-beats, exerting moderate force with your hand

8. Step 15 swaying and shaking: 2 to 3 minutes

9. Tapping the inside of the thigh and calf of Step 14: four 8-beats, tapping the Sanyinjiao point more frequently and exerting moderate force with your hand

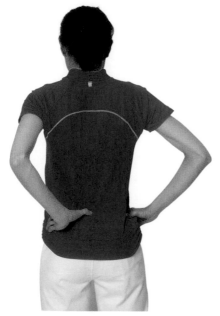

Pinch and rub your Yaoyangguan point.

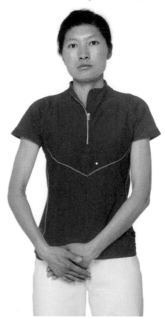

Push and press your abdomen.

Self-Massaging

1. Pinch and rub acupuncture points, including the Shenshu point, Qihaishu point, Yaoyangguan point, Baliao points (i.e. eight sacrum holes, including the Shangliao point, Ciliao point, Zhongliao point and Xialiao point), Xuehai point and Sanyinjiao point. 2 to 3 minutes for each point, once to twice a day.

2. Push and press your abdomen: Overlap your palms and place them on your lower abdomen, exerting force around the Qihai point. 100 to 200 circles clockwise and counterclockwise respectively, once to twice a day.

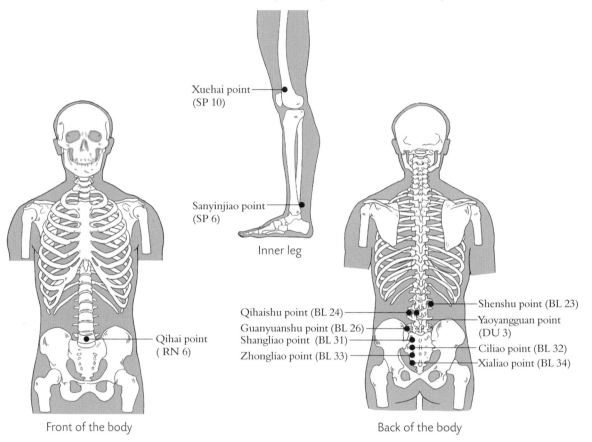

Xuehai point (SP 10)

Sanyinjiao point (SP 6)

Inner leg

Qihai point (RN 6)

Qihaishu point (BL 24)
Guanyuanshu point (BL 26)
Shangliao point (BL 31)
Zhongliao point (BL 33)

Shenshu point (BL 23)
Yaoyangguan point (DU 3)
Ciliao point (BL 32)
Xialiao point (BL 34)

Front of the body

Back of the body

Additional Tips

When menstruating, exposure to wind/cold and humidity should be particularly avoided, and it is best to refrain from intensive labor or exercise. At all times you should pacify your state of mind, relieve mental pressure, and not misuse drugs, particularly antibiotics. You should also refrain from smoking and drinking, and undertake timely systematic treatment for any underlying primary diseases.

Please pay attention to your personal and sexual hygiene, eat light and bland food, and avoid raw, cold, spicy and pungent food. Drink more water. You can increase abdominal exercises and practice lifting from the groin 50 to 100 times before sleep.

18 | Male Sexual Dysfunction

There are many causes of sexual impotence and premature ejaculation, both physical and psychological. These include mental and emotional factors, the health of the relationship, too much or too little sexual activity, drinking alcohol, etc. They are also commonly caused by endocrine dysfunction resulting from diseases, drugs or exposure to radiation.

These diseases should be diagnosed and treated in a timely manner by specialist doctors. Here I make introduction to only the self-healthcare methods that can be applied by patients with functional, not disease-related, causes.

Meridian and Collateral Exercises

Please spend about 20 minutes every day practicing all sixteen steps of the meridian and collateral exercises in Chapter Two. You can also choose the following steps to practice together or separately, once to twice a day, moderately increasing repetitions over time.

1. Step 2 holding a "ball" in a horse-riding stance: four 8-beats
2. Waist rotation of Step 6: four 8-beats. While rotating always place your fists at your waist and back, and support your Guanyuanshu point and various sacrum holes (Baliao points) with the joints of your fingers and your palms so they can be massaged continuously.
3. Hip rotation of Step 6: four 8-beats
4. Ear-lifting of Step 10: left and right side for two 8-beats respectively
5. Push and rub your chest and abdomen of Step 9: four 8-beats, applying gentle force with your hand
6. Tapping the Qihai point and Mingmen point of Step 14: four 8-beats, applying gentle force with your hand
7. Tapping the inside of the thigh and calf of Step 14: four 8-beats, more frequently tapping your Sanyinjiao point and exerting gentle force with your hand
8. Step 13 pushing a "wall": four 8-beats, starting from a high position and gradually transitioning to a full squat
9. Tapping on and along the spine of Step 14: up and down and back and forth, four times of four 8-beats, exerting gentle force with your hand
10. Step 15 swaying and shaking: 2 to 3 minutes

Self-Massaging

1. Pinch and rub your Baihui point, Mingmen point, Shenshu point, Zhishi point, Yaoyangguan points, Baliao points, Zusanli point and Sanyinjiao point. 1 to 3 minutes for each point, once to twice a day.
2. Push and press your abdomen: Overlap the palms and place them at your

lower abdomen. Exert force to your Qihai point, and move counterclockwise for 100 to 200 circles, once to twice a day.

Additional Tips

Take care of your mental health, building up an optimistic outlook and cultivating a harmonious atmosphere at home.

Refrain from smoking and drinking, and maintain a proper diet. Choose moderately-tight underpants and trousers. If these are too tight, it will unfavorably affect blood circulation of the scrotum and interfere with the relief of symptoms.

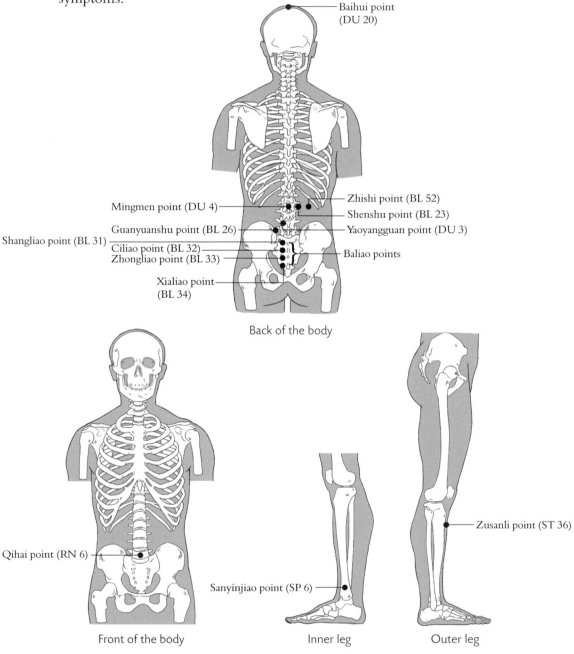

Baihui point (DU 20)

Mingmen point (DU 4)
Zhishi point (BL 52)
Shenshu point (BL 23)
Guanyuanshu point (BL 26)
Yaoyangguan point (DU 3)
Shangliao point (BL 31)
Ciliao point (BL 32)
Zhongliao point (BL 33)
Baliao points
Xialiao point (BL 34)

Back of the body

Qihai point (RN 6)

Zusanli point (ST 36)

Sanyinjiao point (SP 6)

Front of the body   Inner leg   Outer leg

Additional Exercise: Traditional Folk Practice

Efficacy: This practice, called the "iron-crotch skill," can dredge meridians and collaterals closely related to the reproductive and endocrine functions of your body, smooth and clear their qi and blood, and eliminate the symptoms of sexual dysfunction including impotence and premature ejaculation.

Action: Before sleep, lie on your back and relax yourself. Naturally separate your feet. Pull, press and massage in turn with your palm from the Huiyin point in your perineum (the midpoint of the line connecting your anus and the root of your scrotum). Move upward across both sides of the pubis, all the way to the central line of abdomen. Apply continuous slow and gentle force on the left and right side in turn.

You need to repeat this more than 100 times at least, and up to 400 to 500 times when time permits. If you feel warm in your palms, perineum, scrotum and abdomen, then you have achieved the best effect. Please apply suitable force to pull, press and massage for a sufficient amount of time, and do this persistently.

The entire massaging route involves the application of many acupuncture points in your palm, including the Zhongchong point, Laogong point and Yuji point. Rub and press them together with many of the acupuncture points of the scrotum and abdomen, including those that are important for regulating urinary, reproductive and endocrine functions. These include the Shenque point, Qihai point, Guanyuan point, Qixue point, Zhongji point, Dahe point and Jimai point.

Please note that the acupuncture points and the relevant meridians and collaterals affected by the "iron-crotch skill" are the same in males and females. Therefore this method of massaging is suitable for women to practice as well, since it is helpful for regulating female urinary, reproductive and endocrine functions.

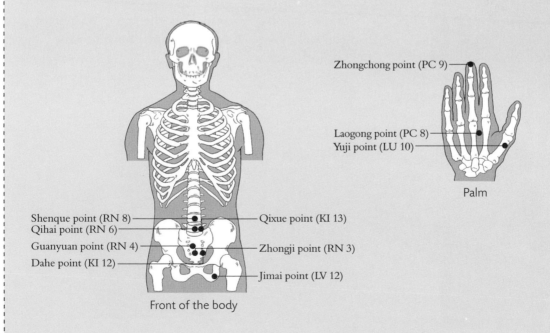

Zhongchong point (PC 9)

Laogong point (PC 8)
Yuji point (LU 10)

Palm

Shenque point (RN 8)
Qihai point (RN 6)
Guanyuan point (RN 4)
Dahe point (KI 12)

Qixue point (KI 13)
Zhongji point (RN 3)
Jimai point (LV 12)

Front of the body

19 | Baldness

A common disease, baldness is closely related to male hormones and endocrine function, heredity, nutrition, mental state and some drug-related factors.

The most common baldness is seborrheic alopecia. Its manifestations include: over-secretion of the sebaceous gland of the scalp; oily scalp; itching; increase of dandruff, thus causing embolism of hair follicle orifices and hyperkeratosis; improper nutrition affecting hair growth; lesion of the hair follicle; and exposure to bacterial infection. Self-healthcare methods can be undertaken in the process of medical treatment.

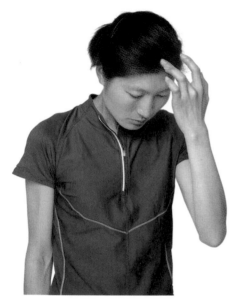

Pinch and rub your Shangxing point.

Meridian and Collateral Exercises

Please spend about 20 minutes every day practicing all sixteen steps of the meridian and collateral exercises in Chapter Two. You can also choose the following steps to practice together or separately, once to twice a day, moderately increasing repetitions over time.

1. Ear-lifting of Step 10: left and right side for two 8-beats respectively

2. Step 8 combing and scraping: four 8-beats

3. Step 7 pinching and rubbing: four times of four 8-beat

4. Tapping on and along the spine of Step 14: up and down and back and forth for four times of four 8-beats

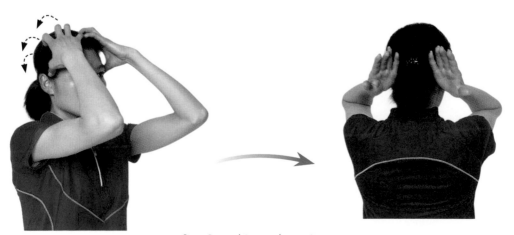

Step 8 combing and scraping

Self-Massaging

Pinch and rub your Baihui point, Shangxing point, Touwei point, Fengchi point, Sanyinjiao point and Shenshu point. 2 to 3 minutes for each point, once to twice a day.

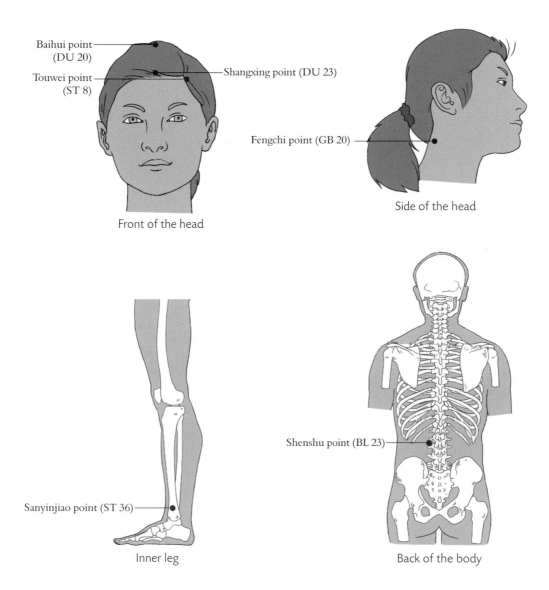

Baihui point (DU 20)

Touwei point (ST 8)

Shangxing point (DU 23)

Fengchi point (GB 20)

Front of the head

Side of the head

Sanyinjiao point (ST 36)

Shenshu point (BL 23)

Inner leg

Back of the body

Additional Tips

Avoid factors that damage your hair, and pay attention to the nutrition and treatment of your hair, e.g. giving up dyeing, heat-straightening and blow-drying. Choose mild liquid shampoo and conditioner.

In addition you should eat mild and bland food, reducing intake of fried and other oily, hot and spicy food. Also important is moderating your work and getting sufficient rest as well as maintaining a good mood.

APPENDICES

Meridian Database: Illustrations, Acupuncture Points and Locations

According to traditional Chinese medicine, acupuncture points are tiny spots where qi and blood are infused in meridians, collaterals and internal organs. They are not only reaction points of diseases, but also stimulation points for acupuncture, moxibustion and other treatment.

Inside the human body, there are 12 "regular" meridian and collateral channels in total. Adding in the Conception Vessel at the front center of the body and the Governing Vessel at the rear center, there are together fourteen meridian and collateral channels. A total of 365 acupuncture points are arranged along them. This book covers the 124 acupuncture points that are often used in the process of tapping meridians and collaterals as a means of self-healthcare.

There are many acupuncture points not included in the fourteen channels that have important efficacies as well as explicit locations and names. These are called "irregular" acupuncture points. This book also introduces three irregular acupuncture points often used in tapping as a means of prevention and treatment.

In naming meridians/collaterals and acupuncture points, this books uses codes from the standard of World Federation of Chinese Medicine Societies—Specialty Committee of Publishers and Editors, namely: abbreviations of meridian/collateral names plus serial numbers.

For acupuncture point names, Chinese pinyin names (transliterated names) and Chinese characters are used. The names often have deep links to Chinese classical culture and profound meanings. By referring to various publications, this book tries to restore the cultural, physiological, diagnostic and therapeutic connotation of original acupuncture point names through translation.

This table also lists the locations of acupuncture points so that readers can find them conveniently. An important means of location is the "cun" measurements of the body. This system is an ingenious way by which anyone can measure and locate acupoints on his or her own body. Since everyone's body is of a different size and shape, using a measurement system specific to the individual makes finding the points easy.

Standard Meridian Abbreviations

Taiyin Lung Meridian of Hand	LU
Yangming Large Intestine Meridian of Hand	LI
Yangming Stomach Meridian of Foot	ST
Taiyin Spleen Meridian of Foot	SP
Shaoyin Heart Meridian of Hand	HT
Taiyang Small Intestine Meridian of Hand	SI
Taiyang Bladder Meridian of Foot	BL
Shaoyin Kidney Meridian of Foot	KI
Jueyin Pericardium Meridian of Hand	PC
Shaoyang Sanjiao Meridian of Hand	SJ
Shaoyang Gallbladder Meridian of Foot	GB
Jueyin Liver Meridian of Foot	LV
Conception Vessel	RN
Governing Vessel	DU
Extra Points of the Head and Neck	EX-HN

The process starts with the measurement of one cun. This is done in two ways:

- Using the width of the distal inter-phalangeal joint of the thumb
- Using the distance between the distal and proximal inter-phalangeal joints of the third (middle) finger.

All other specific measurements are outlined in the diagrams below. When in doubt in measuring, the thumb (1 cun) or the four finger method (3 cun) can always be used.

1 cun

1 cun   1.5 cun   3 cun

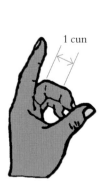
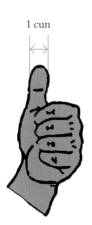
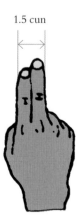
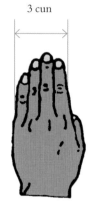

Taiyin Lung Meridian of Hand (LU)

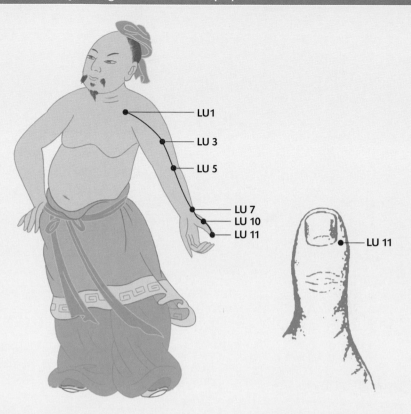

Code	Name of Acupoint		Location
	Pinyin and Chinese	Translation	
LU 1	Zhongfu point 中府穴	Middle Storehouse	6 cun horizontally away from the front central line; in the superior lateral part of the anterior thoracic wall, in the intercostal space of the first rib
LU 3	Tianfu point 天府穴	Celestial Storehouse	On the inner side of the arm, on the radial edge of the biceps brachii; 3 cun below the anterior axillary fold
LU 5	Chize point 尺泽穴	Cubit Marsh	In the cubital transverse crease, and in the depression on the radial side of the biceps brachii
LU 7	Lieque point 列缺穴	Broken Sequence	In the depression of the processus styloideus radii, which emerges after you press down with the tip of the index finger of one hand with the centers of your palms facing inward and the rear parts of your hands, between thumbs and index fingers, crossing each other naturally
LU 10	Yuji point 鱼际穴	Fish Border	In the depression behind the first metacarpophalangeal joint of the thumb
LU 11	Shaoshang point 少商穴	Lesser Stream	0.1 cun beside the corner of the fingernail on the radial side of the thumb

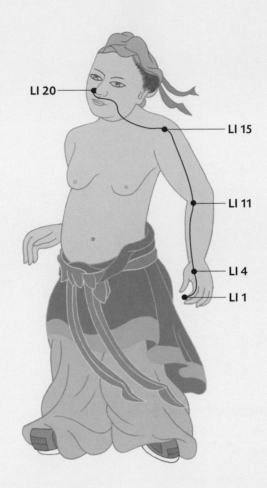

Code	Name of Acupoint		Location
	Pinyin and Chinese	**Translation**	
LI 1	Shangyang point 商阳穴	Yang Stream	0.1 cun beside the corner of the fingernail on the radial side of the index finger
LI 4	Hegu point 合谷穴	Joining the Valley (Union Valley)	At the midpoint between the first and second metacarpal bones on the back of hand
LI 11	Quchi point 曲池穴	Crooked Pond (Pool at the Bend)	On the outer side of the cubital transverse crease of a flexed elbow
LI 15	Jianyu point 肩髃穴	Shoulder Bone	At the center of the deltoid on the outer side of the arm; a depression emerges at the lower back of the shoulder peak when the arm is extended outward
LI 20	Yingxiang point 迎香穴	Welcoming Perfume	0.5 cun beside the wing of nose, in the nasolabial groove

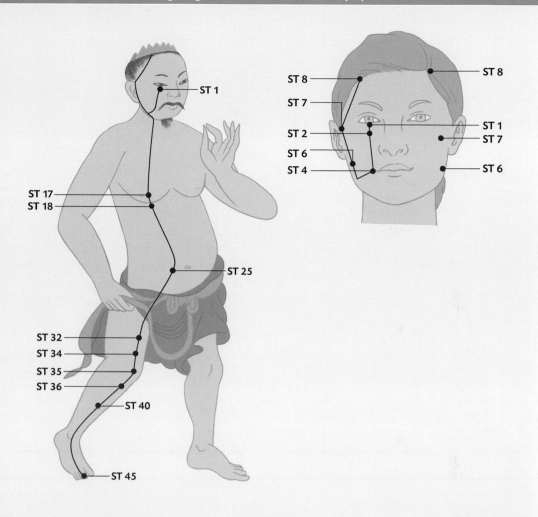

Code	Name of Acupoint		Location
	Pinyin and Chinese	**Translation**	
ST 1	Chengqi point 承泣穴	Tear Container	On the face between the lower edge of the eyeball and eye socket
ST 2	Sibai point 四白穴	Four Whites	In the depression of the orifice under the eye socket, under the central line of the eyeball
ST 4	Dicang point 地仓穴	Earth Granary	0.4 cun beside the corner of the mouth
ST 6	Jiache point 颊车穴	Jaw Chariot (Jawbone)	In the depression one horizontal finger from the upper front of the angle of the mandible; this will crease when the teeth are clenched
ST 7	Xiaguan point 下关穴	Below the Joint	In the depression at the hair line in front of the ear; it can be felt when the mouth is closed and creases when the mouth is open

Code	Name of Acupoint		Location
	Pinyin and Chinese	**Translation**	
ST 8	Touwei point 头维穴	Head Corner	0.5 cun over the hair line at the frontal angle
ST 17	Ruzhong point 乳中穴	Breast Center	At the center of the nipple
ST 18	Rugen point 乳根穴	Breast Root	At the base of the breast under the nipple
ST 25	Tianshu point 天枢穴	Celestial Pivot	2 cun horizontally away from the navel at the center of the abdomen
ST 32	Futu point 伏兔穴	Crouching Rabbit	On the outer edge of the thigh, 6 cun over the patella
ST 34	Liangqiu point 梁丘穴	Beam Hill	On the outer edge of the thigh, 2 cun over the patella
ST 35	Dubi point 犊鼻穴	Calf's Nose	Between the two knee eyes (depressions below the patella of a bent knee)
ST 36	Zusanli point 足三里穴	Three Mile Point (Leg Three Li)	One horizontal finger beside the shin bone, 3 cun under the outer knee eye (the depression below the patella of a bent knee)
ST 40	Fenglong point 丰隆穴	Bountiful Bulge	8 cun over the lateral malleolus
ST 45	Lidui point 厉兑穴	Severe Mouth	0.1 cun from the toenail corner, on the outer side of the second toe

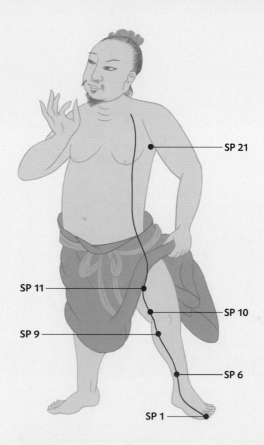

Code	Name of Acupoint		Location
	Pinyin and Chinese	**Translation**	
SP 1	Yinbai point 隐白穴	Hidden White	0.1 cun from the toenail corner on the inner side of the first toe
SP 6	Sanyinjiao point 三阴交穴	Three Yin Intersection	On the rear edge of the shin bone, 3 cun above the ankle
SP 9	Yinlingquan point 阴陵泉穴	Shady Side of the Mountain (Yin Mound Spring)	In the depression on the inner edge of the shin bone by the knee
SP10	Xuehai point 血海穴	Sea of Blood	In the depression at the rear of the patella with bent knee
SP 11	Jimen point 箕门穴	Winnower Gate	6 cun over the Xuehai point
SP 21	Dabao point 大包穴	Great Embracement	In the intercostal space of the sixth rib, along the midaxillary line

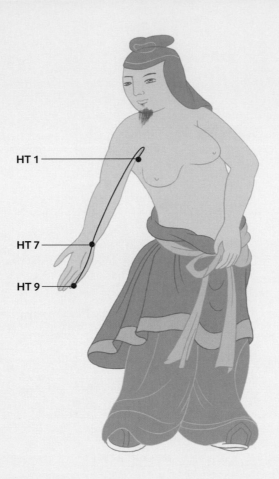

Code	Name of Acupoint		Location
	Pinyin and Chinese	**Translation**	
HT 1	Jiquan point 极泉穴	Highest Spring	At the center of the armpit
HT 7	Shenmen point 神门穴	Spirit Gate	On the ulnar side of the transverse wrist crease, in the depression on the radial ulnar wrist flexor tendon
HT 9	Shaochong point 少冲穴	Lesser Surge	0.1 cun from the inner edge of the fingernail corner of the little finger

Taiyang Small Intestine Meridian of Hand (SI)

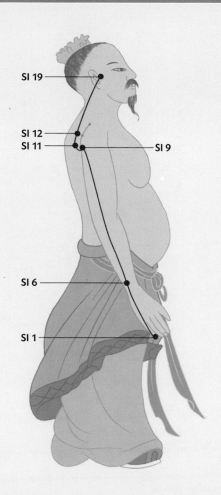

Code	Name of Acupoint		Location
	Pinyin and Chinese	**Translation**	
SI 1	Shaoze point 少泽穴	Lesser Marsh	0.1 cun from the outer edge of the fingernail of the little finger
SI 6	Yanglao point 养老穴	Nursing the Aged	In the depression on the radial side of the near end of the ulna capitulum, on the ulnar side of the back of the forearm
SI 9	Jianzhen point 肩贞穴	True Shoulder	At the lower back of the shoulder joint
SI 11	Tianzong point 天宗穴	Celestial Gathering	In the depression at the center of the shoulder blade
SI 12	Bingfeng point 秉风穴	Grasping the Wind	At the center of the supraspinal fossa of the scapular region, over the Tianzong point; a depression emerges when the arm is lifted
SI 19	Tinggong point 听宫穴	Listening Palace (Auditory Palace)	In front of the antilobium; a depression emerges when the mouth is opened

Taiyang Bladder Meridian of Foot (BL)

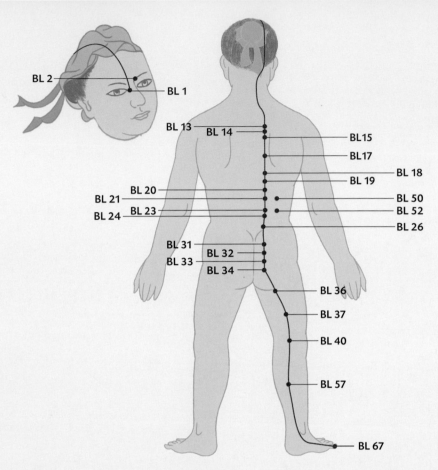

Code	Name of Acupoint		Location
	Pinyin and Chinese	**Translation**	
BL 1	Jingming point 睛明穴	Bright Eyes	In the depression 0.1 cun over the inner corner of eye
BL 2	Cuanzhu point 攒竹穴	Bamboo Gathering	On the edge of the eye socket, on the inner edge of the eyebrow
BL 13	Feishu point 肺俞穴	Lung Associated (Lung Tunnel)	Under the third thoracic vertebra crest of the back, 1.5 cun horizontally away from it
BL 14	Jueyinshu point 厥阴俞穴	Pericardium Tunnel	Under the fourth thoracic vertebra crest, 1.5 cun horizontally away from it
BL 15	Xinshu point 心俞穴	Heart Tunnel	Under the fifth thoracic vertebra crest, 1.5 cun horizontally away from it
BL 17	Geshu point 膈俞穴	Diaphram Tunnel	Under the seventh thoracic vertebra crest, 1.5 cun horizontally away from it
BL 18	Ganshu point 肝俞穴	Liver Tunnel	Under the ninth thoracic vertebra crest, 1.5 cun horizontally away from it

Code	Name of Acupoint		Location
	Pinyin and Chinese	**Translation**	
BL 19	Danshu point 胆俞穴	Gallbladder Tunnel	Under the tenth thoracic vertebra crest, 1.5 cun horizontally away from it
BL 20	Pishu point 脾俞穴	Spleen Tunnel	Under the eleventh thoracic vertebra crest; 1.5 cun horizontally away from it
BL 21	Weishu point 胃俞穴	Stomach Tunnel	Under the twelfth thoracic vertebra crest, 1.5 cun horizontally away from it
BL 23	Shenshu point 肾俞穴	Kidney Tunnel (Sea of Vitality)	Under the second lumbar vertebra crest, 1.5 cun horizontally away from it
BL 24	Qihaishu point 气海俞穴	Sea-of-Qi Tunnel	Under the third lumbar vertebra crest, 1.5 cun horizontally away from it
BL 26	Guanyuanshu point 关元俞穴	Origin Pass Tunnel	Under the fifth lumbar vertebra crest, 1.5 cun horizontally away from it
BL 31	Shangliao point 上髎穴	Upper Bone-Hole	At the rear orifice of the first sacrum, between the posterior superior iliac spine and central line
BL 32	Ciliao point 次髎穴	Second Bone-Hole	At the rear orifice of the second sacrum, below the posterior superior iliac spine
BL 33	Zhongliao point 中髎穴	Central Bone-Hole	At the rear orifice of the third sacrum, below the Ciliao point
BL 34	Xialiao point 下髎穴	Lower Bone-Hole	At the rear orifice of the fourth sacrum, below the Zhongliao point
BL 36	Chengfu point 承扶穴	Support	At the center of gluteal fold
BL 37	Yinmen point 殷门穴	Gate of Abundance	6 cun under the Chengfu point
BL 40	Weizhong point 委中穴	Bend Middle	At the center of the fossa at the midpoint of the transverse crease
BL 50	Weicang point 胃仓穴	Stomach Granary	Under the twelfth thoracic vertebra crest, 3 cun horizontally away from it; 1.5 cun outside Weishu point
BL 52	Zhishi point 志室穴	Will Chamber	Under the second lumbar vertebra crest, 3 cun horizontally away from it; 1.5 cun outside the Shenshu point
BL 57	Chengshan point 承山穴	Supporting Mountain	At the top of the depression between the two muscle bellies of the calves (the depression below the gastrocnemius when the leg is stretched or heel lifted)
BL 67	Zhiyin point 至阴穴	Reaching Inside (Reaching Yin)	0.1 cun on the lateral border of the toenail corner of the little toe

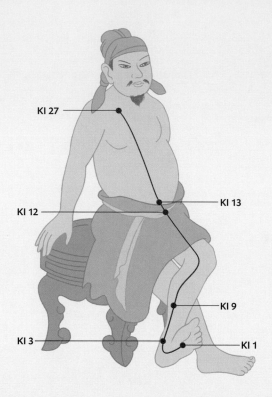

Code	Name of Acupoint		Location
	Pinyin and Chinese	**Translation**	
KI 1	Yongquan point 涌泉穴	Bubbling Spring (Gushing Spring)	In the depression in the front of the sole
KI 3	Taixi point 太溪穴	Bigger Stream (Great Ravine)	In the depression at the midpoint of the inner ankle tip and Achilles tendon
KI 9	Zhubin point 筑宾穴	Guest House	Below the gastrocnemius muscle, 5 cun over the Taixi point
KI 12	Dahe point 大赫穴	Great Manifestation	One finger width horizontally away from the Zhongji point
KI 13	Qixue point 气穴	Qi Hole	One finger width horizontally away from the Qihai point
KI 27	Shufu point 俞府穴	Elegant Mansion (Tunnel Mansion)	2 cun horizontally away from the front central line on the lower edge of clavicle

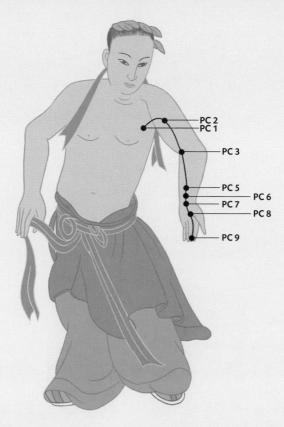

Code	Name of Acupoint		Location
	Pinyin and Chinese	**Translation**	
PC 1	Tianchi point 天池穴	Celestial Pool	3 cun behind the breast and 1 cun under the armpit
PC 2	Tianquan point 天泉穴	Celestial Spring	2 cun under the anterior axillary fold, on the inner side of the arm
PC 3	Quze point 曲泽穴	Crooked Marsh	On the ulnar edge of the tendon of the biceps brachii; in the transverse cubital crease
PC 5	Jianshi point 间使穴	Intermediary (Intermediary Courier)	Between two tendons, 3 cun above the wrist transverse crease; on the palmar side of forearm
PC 6	Neiguan point 内关穴	Inner Gate (Inner Pass)	Between two tendons, 2 cun over the wrist transverse crease
PC 7	Daling point 大陵穴	Big Mound (Great Mound)	Between two tendons at the midpoint of the wrist and palm transverse crease
PC 8	Laogong point 劳宫穴	Palace of Toil	At the middle fingertip of a clenched fist and flexed finger at the center of palm
PC 9	Zhongchong point 中冲穴	Central Hub	At the center of the middle fingertip

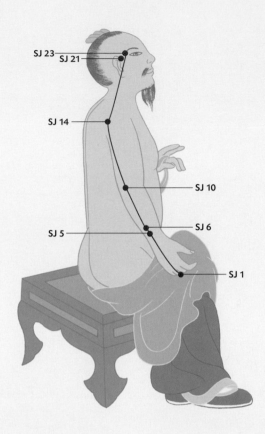

Code	Name of Acupoint		Location
	Pinyin and Chinese	**Translation**	
SJ 1	Guanchong point 关冲穴	Passage Hub	0.1 cun on the outer edge of the fingernail corner of the ring finger
SJ 5	Waiguan point 外关穴	Outer Gate (Outer Pass)	Between the ulna and radius, 2 cun over the wrist-back transverse crease
SJ 6	Zhigou point 支沟穴	Branch Ditch	Between the ulna and radius, 3 cun over the wrist-back transverse crease
SJ 10	Tianjing point 天井穴	Celestial Well	In the depression 1 cun over the tip of the elbow when it is flexed
SJ 14	Jianliao point 肩髎穴	Shoulder Crevice	At the back of Jianyu point; a depression emerges at the lower back of the shoulder peak when the arm is extended outward
SJ 21	Ermen point 耳门穴	Ear Gate	In front of the indentation above the antilobium
SJ 23	Sizhukong point 丝竹空穴	Silk Bamboo Hole	In the depression at the tip of the brow

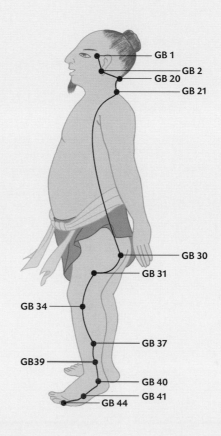

Code	Name of Acupoint		Location
	Pinyin and Chinese	**Translation**	
GB 1	Tongziliao point 瞳子髎穴	Pupil Bone Hole	0.5 cun lateral to the outer canthus of the eye
GB 2	Tinghui point 听会穴	Reunion of Hearing (Auditory Convergence)	In front of the indentation of the antilobium
GB 20	Fengchi point 风池穴	Gates of Consciousness (Wind Pool)	In the depression on both sides of the large tendon behind the nape of the neck, next to the lower edge of the skull
GB 21	Jianjing point 肩井穴	Shoulder Well	At the midpoint of the top of the shoulder
GB 30	Huantiao point 环跳穴	Jumping Circle (Jumping Round)	In the depression on the outer side of the gluteus maximus, on both sides when standing
GB 31	Fengshi point 风市穴	Wind Market	At the middle fingertip when standing upright with hands down; at the central line on the outer edge of the thigh

Code	Name of Acupoint		Location
	Pinyin and Chinese	**Translation**	
GB 34	Yanglingquan point 阳陵泉穴	Sunny Side of the Mountain (Yang Mound Spring)	In the depression at the lower front of the capitula fibula
GB 37	Guangming point 光明穴	Bright Light	On the front edge of the fibula, 5 cun over the lateral malleolus
GB 39	Xuanzhong point 悬钟穴	Suspended Bell	On the front edge of the fibula; 3 cun over the lateral malleolus
GB 40	Qiuxu point 丘墟穴	Wilderness Mound (Hill Ruins)	On the outer side in the depression of the tendon, made when the toe is extended; at the lower front of the outer ankle of foot
GB 41	Zulinqi point 足临泣穴	Above Tears	In the depression on the outer edge of the foot dorsum behind the fourth toe
GB 44	Zuqiaoyin point 足窍阴穴	Portal Yin	On the outer edge of the fourth toe

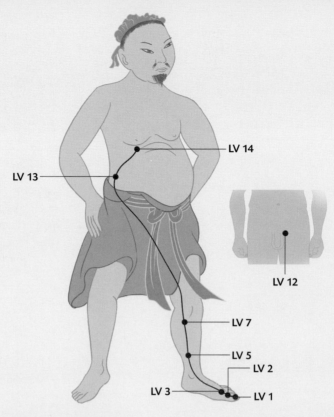

Code	Name of Acupoint		Location
	Pinyin and Chinese	Translation	
LV 1	Dadun point 大敦穴	Large Pile	0.1 cun on the outer edge of the root of the big toenail
LV 2	Xingjian point 行间穴	Travel Between	Between the first and second toe on the foot dorsum
LV 3	Taichong point 太冲穴	Bigger Rushing (Great Surge)	In the depression in front of the junction of the first and second metatarsal bones
LV 5	Ligou point 蠡沟穴	Grind Ditch	5 cun above the inner ankle; at the center of the inner side of shin bone
LV 7	Xiguan point 膝关穴	Knee Joint	1 cun behind the Yinlingquan point
LV 12	Jimai point 急脉穴	Urgent Pulse	On the outer side of tuberculum pubicum; 2.5 cun horizontally away from the front central line
LV 13	Zhangmen point 章门穴	Camphorwood Gate	At the end of the eleventh rib
LV 14	Qimen point 期门穴	Cycle Gate	At the sixth rib under the nipple

Conception Vessel (RN)

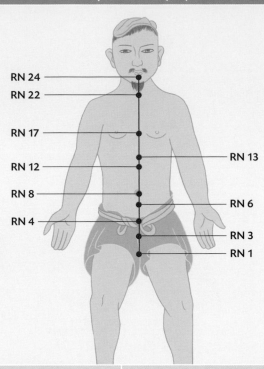

Code	Name of Acupoint		Location
	Pinyin and Chinese	**Translation**	
RN 1	Huiyin point 会阴穴	Meeting of Yin	At the midpoint of the line connecting the anus and scrotum root
RN 3	Zhongji point 中极穴	Central Pole	4 cun below the umbilicus
RN 4	Guanyuan point 关元穴	Gate Origin (Origin Pass)	3 cun below the umbilicus
RN 6	Qihai point 气海穴	Sea of Energy (Sea of Qi)	1.5 cun below the umbilicus
RN 8	Shenque point 神阙穴	Spirit Gate	Navel
RN 12	Zhongwan point 中脘穴	Center of Power (Central Venter)	4 cun above the umbilicus
RN 13	Shangwan point 上脘穴	Upper Venter	5 cun above the umbilicus
RN 17	Danzhong point 膻中穴	Sea of Tranquility (Chest Center)	Parallel with the intercostal space of the fourth rib; at the front central line
RN 22	Tiantu point 天突穴	Heaven Rushing Out	At the center of the suprasternal fossa
RN 24	Chengjiang point 承浆穴	Sauce Receptacle	In the depression at the center of the mentolabial sulcus of the face

Governing Vessel (DU)

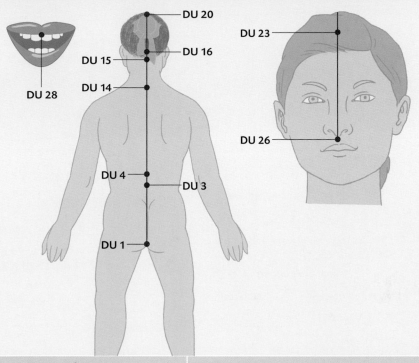

Code	Name of Acupoint		Location
	Pinyin and Chinese	**Translation**	
DU 1	Changqiang point 长强穴	Long Strong	0.5 cun under the tip of the tail bone
DU 3	Yaoyangguan point 腰阳关穴	Lumbar Yang Pass	Under the fourth lumbar vertebra crest
DU 4	Mingmen point 命门穴	Life Gate	Under the second lumbar vertebra crest
DU 14	Dazhui point 大椎穴	Great Hammer	Under the seventh cervical vertebra crest
DU 15	Yamen point 哑门穴	Mute's Gate	0.5 cun over the center of the rear hair line of the neck; under the first lumbar vertebra crest
DU 16	Fengfu point 风府穴	Wind Mansion	1 cun over the center of the rear hair line
DU 20	Baihui point 百会穴	One Hundred Meeting Point	At the center of the skull, over the two ear tips
DU 23	Shangxing point 上星穴	Upper Star	1 cun over the center of the front hair line
DU 26	Shuigou point 水沟穴	Water Trough	In the recessed grove at the center between the nose and upper lip
DU 28	Yinjiao point 龈交穴	Gum Intersection	At the junction between the lip frenum and upper gingival; in the upper lip

Extra Points of the Head and Neck (EX-HN)

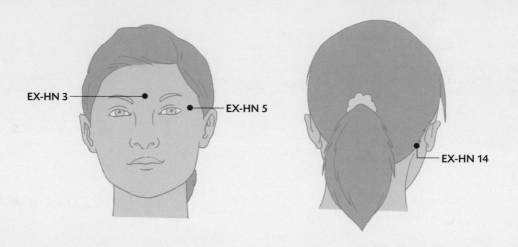

Code	Name of Acupoint		Location
	Pinyin and Chinese	**Translation**	
EX-HN 3	Yintang point 印堂穴	Hall of Seal	At the midpoint of the line connecting the two brows
EX-HN 5	Taiyang point 太阳穴	Temple	In the depression about 1 cun behind the space between the outer tip of the brow and outer eye corner
EX-HN 14	Yiming point 翳明穴	Bright Screen	1 cun behind the depression between the angle of the mandible and mastoid process; behind the earlobe

Index